RECONSTRUCTION OF SOCIAL WORK THROUGH PERSONALISATION

THE NEED FOR POLICY AND PRACTICE SHIFT IN SOCIAL CARE: FAMILY DIRECTED SUPPORT CARE SYSTEMS

FELIX. U. A UGWUMADU

authorHOUSE®

AuthorHouse™ UK Ltd.
500 Avebury Boulevard
Central Milton Keynes, MK9 2BE
www.authorhouse.co.uk
Phone: 08001974150

First published by AuthorHouse 3/10/2011.

ISBN: 978-1-4567-7240-6 (sc)

Abstract

This book is aimed at bridging the gap in the existing literature in the field of social policy for older people; personalisation of services, family reciprocity and education regarding contemporary social care and the social care market in the UK.While there are publications in social inclusion and personalisation, yet, they do not look at the inter-relationships between personalisation of services for older people, family reciprocity and payment to informal family caregivers. In essence, life long learning by service users and their informal carers are lacking and as a result they are not conversant with developments within the system, therefore do not know how to access services within the wider welfare systems. Publications on longevity of care giving to older people, care needs assessment and demographic change also do not focus on life long learning. Thus, this book aims to break new ground by linking these important issues.However, it might be unusual within older people service and long-term care literature to have a focus on the learning needs of a particular population for example; those with long term health and social care problems.

This book has revealed the views of the key stakeholders (service users, family caregivers, social workers, social work managers and councillors) about the potential of family care giving. The majority profess the need for a changed social work practice in order to offer personalisation of services to the growing older people population. In as much as transformation and personalisation are the "buzz words" in social services, yet, many older people would prefer their family members to help them with their social care needs. This view is supported by both practice experiences and empirical research carried out in Essex County Council area of the United Kingdom (Ugwumadu 2010). Thus, the aim of this book is to modernise social work practice in line with the aspirations of the baby boomers that are now entering the social care market. This would provide the opportunity for power balance from the professionals "do it all" to the family members who would carry out assessment of care needs and provide care for older relatives for payment if they wish to.

This book has also highlighted the interrelationships between health and social care for which longevity of care is now prevalence in our society. Presently social policy for older people, in particular the NHS continuing healthcare for older people, is undergoing a considerable paradigm shift in terms of re-thinking core services that have been taken for granted such as collective welfare systems, ability for social inclusion, informal care, education, training, empowerment, and the meaning of recovery from physical disabilities. The re-thinking is accompanied by a slower pace of changes in social care and clinical practices, albeit no less significant, and at times with projects reflecting a leap into the new world of personalisation services.

Glossary

AD	Audit Commission
BV	Best Value
CL	Councillors
CSCI	Commission for Social Care Inspectorate
CSIP	Care Services Improvement Partnerships
DH	Department of Health
DoH	Department of Health
DP	Direct Payments
DWP	Department of Works and Pensions
FG	Family Caregivers
IB	Individual Budgets or Individualised Budgets
IMCA	Independent Mental Capacity Advocate
IPP	Individual Programme Plan
M	Managers
MCA	Mental Capacity Assessment
NHS	National Health Service
NSF	National Service Frameworks
OECD	Organisation for Economic Co-operations and Developments
PCT	Primary Care Trust
RNCC	Registered Nurse Care Contribution
SU	Service Users
UK	United Kingdom
UN	United Nations
UNO	United Nations Organisations

Structures and Diagrams

Contents

ACKNOWLEDGEMENTS

My appreciation goes to; service users, family caregivers, health and social work practitioners, managers and Essex County Councillors that offered practical and policy advice that supported the production of this book.

I extend my special gratitude to my family especially my wife who stood by me and motivated me to write this book.

I owe a great debt to Essex County Council (Social Services); Adults Health and Community Wellbeing who offered me the opportunity of employment through which I developed my practice based-knowledge and experience that guided me to produce this book.

I am grateful to my editors who offered immeasurable support to edit and restructure the content and context of this book.

Introduction

The "Big Society" agenda is aimed to break up public services and devolve their functions to individual service users and their families. Much of what the state currently does, the coalition government of the Conservatives and the Liberal Democrats believe, could be done better by families, volunteers, charities and private enterprise. The function of government should be limited to helping citizens provide for themselves. Thus, the power shift and paradigm change would bring about sustainability of holistic care giving to older people and their families who can concentrate in their caring roles.

In concrete terms, this argument illuminates the need for traditional care systems as an extension of the "Big Society's" social projects and a national citizen service destined to provide security and assurance for later life care. Family care promotes moral courage and accelerated freedom from potential bewilderment. There are possibilities that family members would be there during thick and thin whilst strangers and professionals would go their ways. From professional point of views, something has clearly gone wrong in areas where government and the professionals occupy power therefore, families are relegated, disempowered and the power for decision making on long-term care for older people rested on the professionals.

The aim of this book is to highlight a complementary care model; "personalisation and later life care for older people". The care perspective advocates engaging family members to undertake social care needs assessment and provide care for older relatives for payment. The service framework would not only attract family members with low incomes to participate in the care for their older relatives, but would also rejuvenate the family's norms, values and belief systems of reciprocity.

The ideology points towards a source of social care recruitment and retention, to meet the declining formal health and social care workforce within personal social services for older people.The main explanation of personalisation of services for adult and older people and reciprocal family care giving is provided by materialistic accounts of choice and control, global search for employment, socio-economic circumstances confronting family caregivers, respect and dignity for the cared for person. This provides a meaningful understanding as to why there is a shortage of social care workers, and to an extent, the family care giving. Family participation in care giving and support to family caregivers have received little, if any, analytical attention despite their vital legislative and policy relevance such as the Carers (Recognition and Services) Act (1995), Carers and Disabled Children Act 2000; Carers Act 2007).

Therefore, this book will address some of the issues relevant to adult and older people's services, bearing in mind personalisation and consumerism policy frameworks. For each, the book highlights the advantages of the care model and draws a comparison with the existing care models; individual budgets, managed service/direct provision and direct payments that render neither able to provide a solid understanding of the nature and causes of declining numbers of health and social care workers to assist service users with their care needs (Alcock 1998; Ungerson 1997; Beland 2005; Glennerster 2006; Glendinning et al 2009).

The focus is to introduce a flexible policy framework, a care model for adult and older people where the family caregivers and the state could work collaboratively; ensuring the needs of service users are met cost effectively (Blair 1998a; Kiernan et al 1999; Lewis 2005). This approach is called "swinging social care market" (see detail below). The model would empower the family caregivers to participate in assessment and care giving to older relatives for payment and they would also be offered carers break in addition to avoid care breakdown. The state would only intervene where there are potential care collapsing or abuse of the cared for person. The aim is to introduce this care model within the wider social care market for adult and older people services.

Given the wide-ranging issues that are associated with personalisation and later life care giving, the book will be illustrated in seven chapters:

1. Policy, practice and the political Paradigm.
2. Reciprocal family care systems for older relatives.
3. The need for and potential of a new care model involving payment for family assessment and care giving
4   The stakeholders views
5   Sustainability of Personalisation of services
6   Personalisation beyond informal care systems.
7   Family care giving and the social care market.

Chapter One:
Policy, Practice and the Political Paradigm

Introduction

New Labour's ideology is based on a set of ideas that directs the party's goals, expectation and action to modernise public services whilst, the coalition government of the conservatives and the Liberal Democrats is focused on the "Big Society" agenda. In that respect, ideologies are systems of abstract thought applied to public matters and thus make this concept central to politics. The main purpose behind an ideology is to offer change in society, and adherence to a set of ideas where conformity already exist, through a normative thought process. Thus, the modernisation agenda amongst other ideological commitments of New Labour and the "Big Society" agenda includes: promoting collaboration between agencies; partnership; improving protection and raising standards; delegation of responsibilities to individuals, families, communities and the voluntary sector organisations (DoH 1998a; Lister 2001; Cameron 2010). This chapter willalso discuss: NHS and Community Care Act (1990), modernisation of social services (DoH 1998), personalisation of services (DoH 2005 and 2008), the European context of personalisation of personal social services and the Big Society" agenda (Cameron 2010).

Policy and Contextual Frameworks

Older people, carers, professionals and politicians of different political persuasions have long stuck to the view that independence is a prime goal for care in the community. This is in line with a whole stream of policies and legislation dating back to the 1970s, supporting the development of community care which was based on the premise that it is better to maintain people in their own home (Boyson 1971; Doyal and Gough 1984; DHSS 1989). New Labour government has confirmed this in Modernising Social Services (DoH 1998), the National Service Framework for Older People (DoH 2001a), and Health and Social Care Act (DoH 2001). The

1

gap between policy, legislation and practice is widening (King's Fund 2006; Commission for Social Care Inspectorate 2006 & 2007). Many local authorities prefer residential placement to domiciliary care because it is cheaper and more convenient to co-ordinate costs and management than domiciliary care (Oldman; Wanless Report 2006).

A contrasting perspective from Kontos and Angus (2001), as well as the Commission for Social Care Inspectorate (2006a & 2007), suggested that the delivery of long-term home care was being changed fundamentally from traditional notions of home into labour-intensive nursing/care assistance. It challenged the idea that home, as we are encouraged to understand it, could be maintained under these conditions. We need to consider the role of residential care as part of a broad preventative strategy. It is known that some care packages are complex and could only be met in a residential setting (Lymbery and Butler 2004). This strategy is linked with the aim and objectives of the flexible social care market concept of care in the community. Residential care would only be required as a last option when it becomes apparent that holistic care needs of older relatives can no longer be maintained in the community.

Care in the community has been around for many years, but the Conservative governments in power from 1979 to 1997 strengthened the framework with the NHS and Community Care Act (DoH 1990). The legislation called for the development of the private and voluntary sector in the delivery of social care for older relatives at home. Fowler (1984), Lewis and Glennerster (1996), Land (2004) and Commission for Social Care Inspectorate (2006) called for social services departments to become "enabling" authorities, moving away from delivering services themselves to commissioning and purchasing services from the independent sector. Similarly the Department of Health and Social Security (1981b) recognised that the strength of informal support available to people was often critical to the feasibility and cost effectiveness of community-based packages of care, which depended for success on a high level of commitment from informal carers. This perhaps included the recognition that the contribution of carers was not as cost free as the White Paper "Working for People" (DHSS 1989) had implied (Lewis and Glendinning 1996; Lewis 2004).

Legislative Dimensions
Community Care, Assessment and Care Management
The Working for People guidance (Department of Health and Social Security 1989) and the NHS and Community Care Act (DoH 1990) defined care in the community as services that respond flexibly and sensitively to the needs of individuals and their carers; allow a range of options for

2

consumers; intervene no more than is necessary to foster independence; and concentrate on those with greatest needs. These statements have appeared to emphasised choice and independence, giving older people the opportunity to say where they wish their care to be provided and who is to provide care for them. This implies that community care means providing the right level of intervention and support to enable older people to achieve optimal independence and control over their lives. This would be achievable in a situation where the user is physically able to do so. However, ageing, medical conditions, frailty and sometimes physical disabilities would make it impossible for many of them to achieve the aims of Community Care without adequate support from the family or state (Milner and O'Byrne 2002).

The legislation (the NHS and Community Care Act - DoH 1990) introduced the split between the functions of purchasing and providing care with greater encouragement for the independent sector to participate in care provision (Fowler 1984; Land 2004) This confirmed the framework as: needs assessment must be carried out where it appears to the local authority that any person for whom they may provide or arrange community care services, may be in need of such services. Where services of health or housing may be needed; the local authority should notify them (s.47) and invite their assistance (Griffiths 1988).

A needs-led assessment may identify the users' and carers' needs, but the provision and care was constrained by the resources available to meet their holistic needs (Whitely 1981; Thane 2000). If the resources are not increased, the rationing of resources remains the same as when the process was service-led. Yet, the researcher's observation in his social work practice is that older people have little or no choice of what goes into their care package, the time at which the services are to be provided, the person who delivers it, or how much they receive, and this is reflected in the findings of Glendinning et al (2002) in their previous study.According to the Commission for Social Care Inspectorate (2006) and King's Fund (2006), the mix of services was very limited and older people only had one or two services in the package of care due to the strict Fair Access to Care Matrix (DoH 2002b). This highlighted the contradiction between choices and resource availability within the welfare service and this was one of the gaps that influence assessment and care.

Policy Shift
The emphasis at the present time, in the social care market, is on intensive prevention of admission to hospital or residential/nursing care home. The central plank of both Department of Health and Social Security

(1989) and the NHS and Community Care Act (DoH 1990) were "promoting choices" for care in the community. The question is what happened to clients' choice about where and how community care is provided and who provides it. Has the strategy of avoidable hospital admission, residential care or nursing home been met in practice with adequate resources, sufficient and good enough social workers, social care providers, community nursing/healthcare, to promote the policy emphasis? The answer here may be probably not. Shortage of both carers and assessors is a national problem. Even if the investment had been made, there are limited resources available to meet the needs of the growing older people population (Wanless 2006).

The emphasis on intensive prevention of residential/nursing care placement appears to have changed little in the market (Essex Social Services 2002; Wanless 2006). Due to a higher dependency levels and increased longevity, a large number of older people are being placed in either residential care or a nursing home (Wanless 2006; Commission for Social Care Inspectorate 2006). However, because of a shortage of carers to provide the intensive care packages required by older people in their own home, their holistic care needs are not adequately met as and when necessary. Many of them have to wait for assessment and care which contributes to the frustrations of older people and their families (Essex Social Services (Best Value Report) 2002; Commission for Social Care Inspectorate 2006a, 2007).

From policy and practice perspectives, what would be the psychological and physical effects on older people by placing them into nursing or residential homes? Are the aspirations of older people to be cared for as long as possible in their own home being realised? What happens to those older people with lesser dependency levels who do not meet the Fair Access to Care legislation matrix? The answer to these questions is that older people are still being seen as a homogenous set of users with little or no choice of who provides care to them and or where their care needs could be met (King's Fund 2006; Lewis 2006; Glennerster 2006).

Nevertheless, there is a danger that the value of residential care for some older people will be overlooked in the current debate and they will be driven towards family supported care systems, although staying in the community for as long as possible. If the concept of family care giving is to be achieved, there should be sufficient capacity and resources, with social workers and carers available to ensure continuity of care for older relatives. Residential care should continue to be a viable option, not only for those who would welcome the security, comfort and care offered by good residential care homes, but also a relief and assurance to both the

4

service user and the family who should not be overburdened during the period of care giving (Lewis 1993; Lloyds 2002).

The move towards the private sector was already afoot through changes within the Department of Health and Social Security and funding arrangements to fund nursing and residential placements (Townsend 1983; Wall 1995). This led to a huge increase in the numbers of older people entering private residential care in the 1980s and early 1990s, with a high proportion funded by the Social Security budget without any assessment of needs, unlike those entering local authority homes. The Audit Commission (1986) identified this as a "perverse incentive" towards institutional care. The Griffiths Report recommended a more co-ordinated approach to funding and management of care, with social services departments taking the responsibility for allocation of funds, assessment of need and co-ordination of care. This formed the genesis of needs assessment and funding of social care by social services and modernisation of social services has continued to direct new changes and development in the welfare systems

Modernisation of Services

To deliver these policy frameworks, the government has passed pieces of legislation. For example, the NHS Plan (DoH 2000) indicated the need for providing high quality services to users and also the opportunity for collaboration between health and social care in order to reduce cost and duplication of services. This framework is interrelated and linked with the Community Care (Delayed Discharges) Act (DoH 2003) that requires social services and health to work collaboratively to facilitate rapid discharges from hospital of all people who need social care assistance following their discharge. If any discharge is delayed for reasons that are deemed to be within the control of social services, the hospital must be reimbursed to the extent of £100 per day and £120 in Greater London.

The No Secret Act (DoH 2000) provided the guidance and processes to follow in order to protect and prevent abuse of vulnerable adults. The Act detailed issues that could be assumed as actual or potential abuse: physical, financial, sexual, deprivation and institutional. Social workers are now empowered to investigate; working jointly with Law enforcement agencies in all forms of allegation of abuse and prosecute where possible. On the other hand, The Care Standards Act (DoH 2002a, 2002a) provided the directives, separating out inspection of social services from the provider with the National Care Standards Commission and this led to the establishment of Commission for Social Care Inspectorate (now merged with health inspection agency and renamed Care Quality Commission).

The Care Standards Act provides the opportunity to root out poor quality of care, both in institutional and domiciliary care setting – thus promoting whistle blowing and enhanced social care provision.

Similarly, the Single Assessment Process (2001d) stands out as one of the important policies linked to the ideology of New Labour government. It is aimed towards inter-agency working and to overcome multiple assessments on an individual service user by different agencies. This policy framework provided a one stop assessment process – giving the service users the opportunity to provide historical information about their health and background as deemed appropriate to facilitate individualised care planning without repeating themselves to other agencies (DoH 2001d). Information could be retrieved and upgraded by different agencies as consented to by the service user.

Also featured prominently within the modernising agenda was the National Service Framework for Older People (DoH 2001a), which was intended to provide the basis for inter-agency working between health and social care services for older people. There are four general themes within the National Services Framework for older people, with eight standards being linked to these themes. The policy framework contains some themes and standards that are less directly relevant to social care. For example, standard 4 relates to general hospital care, while standard 5 relates to stroke care.

Equally significant in promoting the modernising agenda is – Intermediate Care (DoH 2002g), which is one of the developments in the delivery of services for older people. Intermediate care is aimed to enable more service users to regain and maintain their independence and also to reduce the numbers of people occupying acute hospital beds. Undoubtedly, intermediate care has made great strides, but needs to move on to the next phase in its development if it is to be fully accepted and realise its potential to transform the way in which services are delivered and the experiences of people who receive those services (DoH, 2002g).

The Modernisation of Social Services has been seen as a vehicle to convey partnership working between agencies in order to promote: consumerism, personalisation of care and cost savings within the wider welfare systems. However, a number of authors such as Glendinning, Powell and Rummery (2002), Leadbeater (2004) and Hasler (2006) have criticised the policy framework for lacking clear guidance on how best to manage resources between agencies. Hudson (2002) highlighted the difficulties of working effectively across professions who use different theory and practice models and values bases. The shift into a more coercive attitude towards partnership development did not sit comfortably between health and social care as the organisations have separate criteria for success, which is also defined and measured in different ways (Callaghan 2003).

Marketisation of Social Care

The agenda for marketisation of social care revisited familiar themes around the enhanced involvement of users in service delivery, upholding choice and control and increasing accountability and developing these by integrating a role for self-organisation and independent living within services. The modernisation of the social care market, drawing on the principle of provider/purchaser split (NHS and Community care Act (DoH 1990), managerialism in welfare services and best value cost effectiveness, provided a focus for delivering social care. Both Conservative and New Labour administrations have pursued these ideologies. It also has included the privatisation of care for older people, raising the issue whether the for-profit sector in indeed likely to be the best option for good quality care, especially for frail older people.

A key feature of marketisation policy is about breaking down large-scale organisations providing social care and using competition to enable exit or choice by service users. The ideological position is to increase flexibility in the social care market as this would bring about equilibrium of demand and supply in the market. Individuals and groups at different positions on the political spectrum have promoted the idea of users' rights to exercise choice in their use of public services. Progressive self-help movements have argued for choice as a means of promoting market-based solutions and curbing the power of the state (Clarke et al 2000; Leadbeater 2004).

Marketisation significantly centred on issues of cost efficiency, consumerism, and responsibilities and cost savings, whereby the allocation of cash (direct payments) rather than services raised concerns as to the accountability of government monies.Marketisation policy clearly presents significant opportunity for delivering personalisation of services through direct payments and individual budgets model and related support structure in the future social care market (Leadbeater 2004; Hasler 2006). According to Zarb and Nadash (1994) and Hasler (2000, 2006), they argued that direct payments is around 40% cheaper than direct provision. New Labour government assured in its positioning of direct payments and individual budgets as part of a wider marketisation of social care, established initially through the 1990 Community Care Act. This framed the market as an instrument for accessing choice and diversity in social care provision through the development of local care markets (Hasler 2006).

The central doctrines for New Labour government' agenda are: a focus on managerialism not policy and on performance appraisal and efficiency; the disaggregating of public bureaucracies into agencies which deal with each other on a user-pay basis; the use of quasi-markets and contracting out to foster competition; cost-cutting; and a style of management which emphasises, amongst other things, out-put targets, limited-term contract, monetary incentives and freedom to manage (Hood 1991; Osborne and Gaebler 1992; Leadbeater 2004). These ideological policy frameworks are fundamental principles behind this New Labour government's agenda to enhance the welfare systems. Marketisation approach is claimed to offer the opportunity to deliver the personalisation agenda and to maintain cost effective social care.

However, many people would disagree with this position on the grounds illuminated below. For example, changes in delivering personal social services are accompanied by an increasing tendency to define home care intervention in terms of narrow tasks. This has resulted in complaints of unmet needs and lack of opportunities for more generalised social interaction between carers and service users (Sale and Leason 2004). The continuous changes within social services' policy and practice have influenced social work practice and social care delivery. According to Morris (1993a) and Glendinning et al (2002), changes in policy meant that social workers were no longer in a position to uphold social work ethical practice, but had to participate in a policy that deprived users of their rights and choices, as outlined in the National Health Services and Community Care Act (DoH 1990).

It is also possible to see the Community Care (Direct Payments) Act (DoH 1996 a & b), and the Carers and Disabled Children Act (DoH 20001 b) as an attempt by government to promote a distorted and flawed notion of empowerment by exit, shifting responsibilities to users. The aim was to control and reduce an escalation of public expenditure. In such a service, Leece (2000) claimed that it would be left to local authority social services departments to balance the books and reconcile the very real demand for direct payments with already stringent budget constraints. Pearson (2004a, b and 2006) noted the contradiction and tension between the legislation and practice.

New Labour has largely intensified the marketisation approach as the basis of their broader modernisation programme in social care with its increasing focus on personalisation services (Leadbeater 2004): Personalisation is a very potent but highly contested and ambiguous idea that could be as influential as a privatisation was in the 1980s and 1990s in reshaping public provision (Leadbeater, 2004 p 18).

Personalisation of Services

Leadbeater (2004) as well as Care Services Improvement Partnership (2006) explains the history and rationale behind the personalisation of services, which was introduced in "Putting People First: a shared vision and commitment to transformation of adult social care". "Putting People First" notes other key concepts for personalisation: independent living, participation, control, choice and empowerment; also the link with individual or personal budgets. It notes examples of good practice on specific issues in relation to implementing personalisation of social care for older people. It is about promoting a positive culture for introducing individual budgets or direct payments by engaging older people on how individual budgets could make a difference to them and how they could choose to use their Individual Budgets (DoH 2005).

Personalisation is seen as one of the pathways to deliver the modernisation agenda and Hunter and Ritchie (2007) observed that personalisation is about putting service users at the heart of public services, enabling them to become participants in the design and co-production of services. They concluded that social care will be more effective and quality of care assured. Personalisation has the potential to reorganise the way public services are created and delivered to users/potential users within the wider welfare systems. This means personalisation would offer modest modification from mass produced social care, which is common to direct provision, or managed service by social services. Personalisation could just mean more 24/7 hours services, booked appointments and timely access to standardised services (Care Services Improvement Partnership 2006). Personalisation is about giving people much more choice and control over their lives, and goes well beyond just giving personal budgets to those eligible for social care.

According to Leadbeater (2004) as well as Hunter and Ritchie (2007), the personalisation agenda is aimed to achieve five distinctive benefits to service users for example: 1) It would sustain support for the existing services by making them more personalised. 2) Personalisation could also mean giving users the opportunity to participate in navigating their way through services once they have got access to them. 3) The service users make the decision on how best to utilise their budget and chose who provides care to them. 4) Personalisation empowers the users to be co-designers and co-producers of their services. Social workers would only help to build up the knowledge and confidence and they are left to carry on the responsibility on their own. 5) Personalisation has the hallmark of self-organisation: the public good emerging from within society, in part, through the way that public policy shapes behaviours and values in society.

However, for personalised care to be fully integrated within the wider welfare system, personalisation of services will have to be defined in terms of: ensuring quality; meeting people's needs; promoting independence; providing choice and control; and supporting the whole community and family involvement. Hunter and Ritchie's (2007) assertion is that while commissioning is improving, the following must be borne in mind: involving the public and people who use services; encouraging flexibility and innovation; and working out what effective joint commissioning will look like in the future. While personalised services have the potential to empower the service user, there is an increasing awareness of how vulnerable people might be abused when using the services obtained through direct payments. Personalisation and co-production exposes social workers to uncertainty and challenges, which have to be balanced by strong support and supervision (Leadbeater 2004; Hunter and Ritchie 2007).

Health and social work practice have identified four areas of policy and practice that demonstrate how the drive to personalise services has exposed tensions between old and new social care legislation. First, direct payments are currently constrained by the Health and Social Care Act 2001, section 51 - that is, until an amendment in the Health and Social Care Act 2008 comes into force. Second, on individual budgets: a client who decides not to take all or part of an individual budget as a direct payment is currently unable to decide how this can be spent. Third, on self-assessment, the NHS and Community Care Act (1990) require the local authority to assess a person's need for community care services. Lastly, on preventive services, the Fair Access to Care Services has influenced the potency of preventive services in many areas for example social services tend to provide care with critical and substantial needs. Personalisation is the mechanism through which to deliver direct payments and individual budgets within the welfare systems (Lister 2001; Pearson 2004a; DoH 2005, 2008; Glendinning 2008 et al).

Direct Payments

Direct payments have been seen as a means to increase people's direct control over the way in which they want to live their lives. The Community Care (Direct payments) Act (1996) gave local authorities across Britain the power to make cash payments to disabled people (Hasler 2000 and 2006). Initially this was restricted to people under the age of 65 with physical and sensory impairments, learning disabilities and mental health problems, but was later amended in 2000 to include older people, 16-17 years old and parents of disabled children (Maglajcic et al 2000; Leadbeater 2004). The legislation established eligibility for direct payments through local authority care procedures, thereby enabling access through the same assessment system as directly provided social services. This has distinguished policy from other examples of direct payments for disabled people such as the Independent Living Fund, which is paid through central government funding to a designated charity, and social security payments such as the Disability Living Allowance (Hasler and Zarb 2000; Glendinning et al 2000 a & b).

Over the past few years, New Labour has clearly set out its support for the ethos of direct payments as a model of service provision in order to achieve the personalisation agenda in social care. New Labour clearly envisaged direct payments as the mainstream option within community care services (Lewis 2002; Hasler 2006). Some of the recent policy documents have linked in with an independent living discourse through pledges to reconfigure the wider network of support for disabled people. At the same time, direct payments remains lodged within a broader welfare market agenda, with this rhetoric reconstructed around a new focus on the personalisation of care (Leadbeater 2004). Direct payments was implemented with the view to address some of the criticism of managed services within the welfare systems, and the new public management approach was envisaged as a focus to achieving the 3 Es (economy, efficiency and effectiveness) in the social care market.

Direct payments gives users control over money spent on meeting their community care needs rather than receiving services arranged for them by their local authority. They have therefore become an important social policy through their capacity to empower service users through the receipt of a cash sum funded by the state to but specific service (Campbell 1996; Leadbeater 2004). However, take-up of direct payments across Britain was especially poor during the initial period of implementation, yet the government underlined its commitment to the policy through a series of legislative changes (Pearson 2004b; Riddell et al 2005). The early shift in June 2000 to grant older people over the age of 65 access to a direct payment was followed up by a comprehensive set of reforms outlined in the legislation. Central to these changes was the enforcement of a mandatory duty placed on all local authorities to offer direct payments to all eligible groups from June 2003 (Pearson 2006).

The rationale is to extend choice to the user who will have greater control over their care resources. Thus, the user would take on the responsibilities of advertising for and recruiting their own personal assistant independently from social services. The user would be the legal employer of the personal assistant and as a result would be liable for paying their wages, drawing up the contract of employment, ensuring health and safety and paying the national insurance contribution of their care assistant. The service user is mandated to account to social services for the expenditure incurred for care giving on a quarterly basis, which gives social services the opportunity to monitor the care package and cost of care delivery (Community (Direct payments) Care Act - DoH 1996).

Whilst direct payments do bring a number of real advantages for users (Hasler 2006), there are a number of limitations and contradictions that social workers and users are unclear about. According to Glasby and Glasby (1999), Glasby and Littlechild (2000 a & b) and Sale and Leason (2004) some older people expressed concerns about taking up direct payment because of their inability to advertise for personal assistants and be held responsible as a legal employer. They could also be accountable for any breach of employment laws and this presented some dilemma for development and acceptance of direct payments against direct provision.

Another barrier to direct payment was that, whilst some social workers were enthusiastic about the scheme, others felt constrained by their workloads and were concerned about how best to convey the scheme to service users. The lack of designated caseworkers from independent living advocacy meant that this task often fell on social workers or family members who lacked the knowledge and experience of direct payments (Leece 2000). According to Leece, this difficulty meant that direct payments were exposed to abuse by a minority of users, family members and social workers. Hasler (2000) noted that some social workers were unsure about their role when assessing whether someone was willing and able to take part in the scheme, and as a result social workers were not keen for direct payments

There appeared to be tensions between promoting empowerment versus protecting users against abuse. Abuse can take different forms such as financial, negligence and physical and the question is who would monitor direct payments and make sure that personal assistants were not abusing the cared for person. Direct payments appear to be complex and costly in terms of the availability and level of services on offer (Hasler and Zarb 2000; Hasler 2000). According to Hasler, older people valued the freedom of the family care system on offer and preferred their family to manage their care package rather than a stranger. Some carers felt that the scheme was a means to enhance their own choice and control, raising questions as to who was going to benefit most from the scheme.

Despite early enthusiasm and the ongoing contribution of a number of key authorities such as Essex and Cheshire, the implementation of direct payments has been uneven although some progress has been made both at national and regional levels (Sale and Leason 2004). Whilst the number of direct payments has being increased in every category, this increase was far from uniform across council areas. In every category some council reported fewer payments than for the previous year, whilst some had made large increases. Overall, the wide range of direct payments proportionate to population indicated that in every category there was considerable unrealised potential for direct payments in the majority of local council areas. In view of the inadequacies of direct payment and the failure to achieve its potential, New Labour government legislated and implemented individual budget with the aim to address the shortfalls of direct payment scheme.

Individualised Budgets

The idea behind individual budgets is to enable people needing social care and support to participate and decide the nature of the services they need. The individual budgets project is led by the Department of Health in partnership with Communities and Local Government and the Department for Work and Pensions (DoH 2005 a & b and 2006). Individual budgets, sometimes called Individualised budgets or personal budgets. It covers a multitude of funding streams besides adult social care, such as Supporting People, Disabled Facility Grant, Independent Living Funds, Access to Work and Community Equipment Services (Lewis 2002; DoH 2005 & 2006; DWP 2005, 06).

Individualised budget or cash for care is a new government initiative that would complement the conventional service frameworks. It was anticipated that the framework would be implemented nationally in September 2009. It is designed to bring about independence, flexibility and choice for people receiving care. The scheme would give service users a full understanding of the finance that is available; in order to empower them to take control and make decisions about the care they receive. The main idea behind an individual budget is to put the person who is supported or who is given services in control of deciding what support or services they get (DH 2005b).

It is envisaged that individual service users would be empowered to participate in making decisions about their care package and that users would be recognised as the people best placed to understand their own needs and how to meet them. The aim is that individual budgets would be flexible enough to allow people who are satisfied with existing services to keep these, but also to give people a range of options for building up more individually tailored support using direct payments and other routes (DoH 2005a & b). However, as observed by Leabeater (2004) and Hasler (2006), use of individual budgets or self directed care would be difficult to achieve by the majority of older people due to some chronic medical conditions, disabilities and frailty.

The key differences between direct payments and individual budget or cash for care is that a family member living in the same household as the client could be paid for providing care for their older relative as the last resort where other options had failed. Approval for this decision would not be referred to a senior social services manager. Allocated funds could be used to buy any support service appropriate to enhance independence and wellbeing, irrespective of the care plan agreed during the assessment of needs by a social worker (DoH 2005).

Carers' Views of Individual Budgets

Evaluation of the individual budgets pilot by Glendinning and Rummery (2008) revealed that when carers of people with individual budgets were compared with carers of people using direct payment or direct provision, the findings indicated that individual budgets have potential over the existing care models. A significant number of carers reported that individual budgets would improve their quality of life with social care outcomes. Individual budgets assessment and support planning offered more opportunities for carers' involvement than the existing care pathways and social care practice. The pilot revealed that carers of individual budget users were significantly more likely than carers of people in receipt of conventional services to have been involved in planning the user's support arrangements. Carers were also satisfied with the value of the potential care model and how it was being paid. However, there was no statistically significant difference in carers' satisfaction with individual budget support planning than the existing care pathways.

This may reflect both the different support needs of each group and user group-related differences in social care practice (Glendinning and Rummery 2008). Carers of older people were more likely to report that their own needs and circumstances had been taken into account in the service user's individual budget assessment and service planning, compared with previous experiences of direct provision or direct payments. The findings suggested that individual budgets generated more work for carers in managing paperwork and on-going support arrangements. Carers reported uncertainty over how the individual budgets could be used, the management of under spent individual budgets, and problems with support plans that failed to materialise (Glendinning and Rummery 2008).

Practitioners may need to balance more effectively the needs and interests of service users and carers. Greater clarity and consistency are needed, including payments for carers in the individual budgets of service users, the conditions attached to such payments, and the interaction between such payments and other entitlements such as carer grant payments. Further research is needed on the impact of individual budgets on different groups of carers. Personalisation of services such as direct payments and individualised budget scheme is not only common to the English local authorities. Many other European countries now offer similar schemes within their social care market.

European Context of Personalisation

This section aims to compare and contrast England with some European countries' experiences of personalisation of personal social services such as direct payments, cash for care and individual budgets. The comparison helps to examine the English local authorities' policy, practice, and identifying gaps in service as well as good practice that could be developed and promoted as a core service framework within the wider social care market. Personalisation of services has become a policy focus to many European Community countries and this has been commented by a number of authors such as Wiener et al (2003), OECD (2005), Breda et al (2006) and Glendinning et al (2009):

The primary objective of personalisation of service is to provide financial support for the service users to help meet additional costs of needing care. In other instances cash for care or individual budget or direct payment aims at offering service users consumer-style choice and control over their care needs. These measures differ widely in terms of client groups, eligibility criteria, interactions with formal caregivers, payment levels and whether they are means tested (Glendinning et al 2000 and 2009, Breda et al 2006). The impact on carers also varies, depending local labour market, the availability of formal long-term care providers, and critically important, social attitudes toward the roles of families in caring for older relatives. In practice, instead of receiving direct services provision from local authority, service users can choose to receive a personal budget of an equivalent value to purchase care themselves, either from a provider agency, family members or by directly employing a carer. There is increasing interest in service user directed cash for care schemes as a means of promoting personalisation of care, choice and flexibility in long-term care; such schemes exist in many European countries such as the

UK, the Netherlands, Austria, Belgium, Finland and Sweden (Winener et al 2003; Glendinning et al 2009).

The level of personal budget is usually calculated by multiplying the number of hours of care needed against an hourly rate, usually at the legal minimum wage, therefore in principle offering appropriate economic rewards for care giving. According to Breda et al (2006), carers that are employed in this way report increased feelings of obligation and difficulties in negotiating time off. Consequently, the total value of the care provided usually far exceeds the payment received (Breda et al 2006; Hasler 2006). The reality of the caregiver's income depends on continuing good relationships between employer and employee. Caregivers are also financially vulnerable if the older relative dies or, admitted into hospital or, long-term care. According to Glendinning et al (2009) and Breda et al (2006), personal budget or cash for care may attract new family members, such as newly retired relatives into care work. However, caregivers employed by personal budget holders occupy a marginal position between the formal and informal care workforce; formal training or career advancement schemes are very rare.

In Holland, Denmark, Sweden and Finland, older people are permitted to receive personal budgets with which to purchase care (Coolen and Weekers 1998; Leece 2000). In order to prevent fraud, an independent body administers users' control of the selection of carers while the user controls the money for their personal assistant. Coolen and Weekers (1998) noted a number of financial and social barriers for example, difficulties in establishing personal budgets for older people who use the scheme. Barriers relating to employment rights of caregivers have contributed to some of the difficulties in implementing and smooth running of the scheme. There was also professional opposition from trades' union and formal service providers who felt that the alternative care model of direct provision threatens the job security of social care workers and the profitability of provider agencies.

In Germany, the user's eligibility for social insurance fund is determined by medical assessment and allowances are calculated on the basis of a pre-set national table of needs and cost per hour, and users without medically linked needs would not qualify (Halloran 1998). In Germany, Denmark and France, users are only allowed to purchase care from approved providers and not from family members. The Scandinavian countries such as Sweden and Finland tend to issue vouchers to users for their care to enable them to purchase from the public, but not from family members. English local authorities provide individuals with cash payments; although the service cannot be purchased from the family, apart from in exceptional circumstances, and funding has to be approved by a chief officer of social services.

Research commissioned by the European Association for Care and Help at Home suggested that, the shift towards cash for care was the result of a series of parallel developments that included: 1) the growing demand for care and the fact that available care provided by the welfare system cannot meet new needs. 2) Pressure, especially from organisations of disabled people and Age Concern, who are uncomfortable for the government to ignore as this could have some political ramifications. 3) Accommodating a new service framework, which would produce cheaper and better service and not rely solely on direct provision, which does not give users wide ranging choice and control of their care package? 4) Enhancing a political wish to let people stay longer in their own homes instead of more expensive institutions (Halloran 1998; Lewis 2006 a & b).

The European Association of Care Help at Home (Coolen and Weekers 1998) study concluded that personalisation of services such as direct payments were a good development in the social care market, but sounded a note of caution in that care allowances were practical and useful for certain categories of service users. Those who could handle the responsibilities were, as a rule, positive about this innovation (Leadbeater 2004; Breda et al 2006 and Hunter and Ritchie 2007). For those who had a care allowance, it was important to have recourse to an informal network or to a formal agency to help when there were problems. Care allowances were not a good way of helping the frail or confused and isolated older people who live by themselves.

Cash for care models do little to bridge the boundaries between informal care and formal labour market participation, for example by explicitly encouraging caregivers to retain contact with the labour market while caring. According to Wiener et al (2003) and Breda et al (2006), there is also little evidence of measure to formalise the skills acquired in informal care giving as potential assets for future employment, even where caregivers have previously been employed by cared for person holding a personal budget. Equally, all the cash for care models offer low levels of financial reward in comparison to the actual level of care provided. This even where hourly payment rates are at or above the legal minimum wage; the total volume of care provided usually far exceeds the hours that are actually paid for.

Comparative Conclusion

The comparative analysis above provided a learning opportunity both to practitioners and policy makers within social policy for older people in the European community. Each of the sampled European countries used personalisation - direct payments, cash for care and individual budgets differently and there was no uniformity in approach (Halloran 1998, Leece 2000; Glendinning et al 2000; Glendinning 2009). The English authorities' model of direct payments and individual budgets had a hallmark of personalisation policy framework (Leadbeater 2004; Hasler 2006). Assessment is based on social model of care, cash payment is given directly to the user based on assessed needs, and the money could be used to buy care or equipment depending on needs. The user has the flexibility to exercise choice and control, recruiting and employing their own personal assistance without state interference. The service user may be supported by family members if unable or, can employ an expert who would assist to manage the scheme, and they have the overall decision-making regarding their care (Hasler 2006, Pearson 2004, 2006).

In contrast, the other European countries adopted what is similar to indirect payments in England (Wiener et al 2003; Hasler 2006). For example, in Holland, users have limited opportunity to administer direct payments as an agency is appointed by local authority to recruit carers and manage the cash payments on their behalf. In Germany, qualification for cash for care is determined by medical conditions and medical model of assessment and services are offered through appointed agencies. In France and Germany, services can only be purchased through approved providers, while in Scandinavian countries; users are given vouchers to buy their care from the public, but not from their family members. Users of cash for care in England have greater opportunities and, are empowered to exercise greater choice and control than the European service users of the schemes.

In Finland cash for care is awarded on the bases of an older people's care needs but is paid to directly to the caregiver, who contracts with the municipality to provide an agreed level of care according to the care plan. The majority of the caregivers employed in this way are spouses or other close relatives and a third are aged 65 and over. Levels of payment to carers are lower than the value of formal home care services, they offer no incentive to continue care giving, but are believed to encourage caregivers to continue their existing care giving responsibilities (Breda et al 2006; Glendinning et al 2009). In Austria, recipients of cash for care are likely to use the fund to support family caregivers; professional families are more likely to use it to employ live-in-carers through the grey labour market.

In both instances, the low level of the cash for care institutionalises care giving as woman's work (Kreimer 2006)

Therefore, the policy frameworks of cash for care would enhance modernisation agenda in the wider welfare systems. It is in principle possible for cash for care recipients to use some formal services, which helps to relieve the burdens on family caregivers, given changes within the family units and demographic changes (Pearson 2006; Kreimer 2006; Hunter and Ritchie 2007; Glendinning et al 2009).

The Big Society Agenda

The Big Society is at the heart of traditional Conservatives party's suspicion of public services run centrally from number ten Dowining Street, deemed inefficient at best, counter-productive at worst. The welfare state, in this view, is a bureaucracy governed by targets and rules that cannot adapt to the real-life complexity of social and political breakdown. As a result, some problems get worse: fathers are discouraged from living with the mothers of their children by a benefits system that rewards single parents; the unemployed do not seek jobs because they are better off claiming to be incapacitated by sickness (Cameron 2010). The aim of the coalition government is to overhaul the welfare system and appotion responsibilities to communities and individuals to run their affairs with minimum interference by the state.

The coalition government at present is not consistent to distinguish his Big Society idea from a conventional Thatcherite attack on the state that would leave people to sink or swim, depending on whether they have the good fortune to live somewhere with good economic prospects. However, the Conservative party's manifesto gives meagre reassurance on that point. Where the state is purported to have failed, voluntary action is supposed to come to the rescue, but the method for harnessing that charitable impetus turns out to be mere exhortation – a promise to encourage people to make volunteering something they do on a regular basis. That is not a convincing alternative to the deep national budget deficit.

There is merit in some of the coalition government of the Conservatives and the Liberal Democrats' critique of the state and the aspiration to think imaginatively about reform is laudable. Something has clearly gone wrong in areas where government is the only employer and in families where, for successive generations, benefits have been the only source of income.

Thus, that doesn't mean the solution lies in a sudden government retreat. The transition from state dependency to self-sufficiency must be carefully managed if it is not deplorable and inhumane to users of

19

public services. It will take time and resources. The coalition government might prefer that investment come from volunteers and businesses, and if it wants the job done it will still need to hold them to account and give them money.

The relationship between society and government is not a zero-sum game. It does not always follow that more of one necessitates less of the other. That the Conservatives party seems to believe it does indicates the persistence in their ranks of an ideological prejudice against all state intervention. Many people from different works of life might agree with the coalition government that public spending has run out of control under New Labour government. As it happens, New Labour's own budget puts an abrupt stop to that, stripping nearly 12% from departmental budgets over the last parliament. Government will regardless of who is in power, get smaller. It is peculiar that the Conservatives chose to make that the defining goal of their manifesto, especially when the proposals they have to ease the pain from cuts are so paltry.

The focus for the coalition government is to fulfill an ambition much cherished by the Conservative party in the past which is about cutting back the state without inflicting the social cost that was the price of the same policy in the 1980s. The Big Society model achieves that alchemy. It contains some decent notions, but they quickly fray when stretched into an overarching philosophy. The characteristics of the big society are deely rooted in Britain's history, which enhanced psychosocial wellbeing of the less affluence in society. For example, the great charitable hospital of the 19th century, the municpal aid organisations that provided millions of manual workers with helthcare and unemployment benefits before Lloyd George's National Insurance Act and the extraordinary levels of charitable giving and civic activisim that chractarised Victorian Britian. The Big Society is not a new ideological policy framework, these things happened in the past when Britain was poorer than what it is today.

The Big Society tends to convince the public that the government is unable to overlook the nation's wellbeing as it done since the National Assistance Act (1947) when Beveridge declared war on poverty. This is ultimately the political point of the Big Society agenda: people have become so reliant on government doing things for them and it wants to roll back the state and delegate responsibilities to individuals, communities and voluntary sector organisations. It is anticipated that the private and voluntary sector organisations would fill the gaps, but the adjustment and the process would be painful and the politics of the situation impossible.

Conclusion

This chapter has revealed how the welfare system functions, but failed to illuminate the prominence given to: the economic wellbeing of the family caregivers; gender division of labour, and the role of women in providing welfare services for older people. The reappraisal of the present ideologies noted similarities and differences between the New Right and New Labour's modernisation agenda and then highlighted a number of issues that restricted older people's choices: inter-dependency; access and ability to function well as consumers within the social care market. However, the present family units are smaller, yet traditional family care systems still has a place in our society today and in the future and are still capable enough to support the fragile welfare service. The chapter is privileged to highlight the inconsistencies between the policies and legislative frameworks and how the family members have not been included in making long-term strategic decision about social care for their older relatives. The standpoint for the service framework is that the family and the older relative would jointly have the opportunity to undertake holistic care needs assessment and family caregivers would be paid for care giving to older relatives if they wished to provide care. The value base of the care model is that the family would play a pivotal role advocating the best interest of their older relative's long-term care, working in partnership with social workers.

Chapter Two:
Reciprocal Family Care Systems for Older Relatives

Introduction

The ideological position of this framework is located within the traditional family care model, where the family members are able to uphold their values and belief systems and are capable to exercise choice and control over their functional activities of daily living. In this context, family refers to both blood relatives and to non-related significant family friends or neighbours. Even without this extended definition, the term family contains a bewildering diversity of the meaning. These relatives may have no common purpose or views in relation to the older relative's best interest, yet they try to come together in times of family difficulties to support one another in order to avert family breakdown (Young and Willmott 1957; Finch 1995, 1989). Nevertheless, the experience and views of some family members are often not sought for and therefore unknown or they are ignored by the professionals or decision makers (Carers National Association 2001). This limitation tends to deprive some family members the opportunity to partake in decision making about their older relative's long-term care needs. This chapter is illustrated in three sub-sections: dimensions of family care giving, nature of family care giving and welfare state and changing family unit.

Dimensions of Family Care Giving

The provision of assistance and support by one family member to another is a regular part of family interactions and is a pervasive activity in most families (Burgess 1960; Townsend 1983; Phillipson et al 2001). Care giving due to old age, frailty and disability represents something that in principle is not very different from traditional tasks and activities undertaken for family members. This is especially true for women who across cultures have traditionally shouldered a disproportionate amount of family care giving responsibility (McGoldrick 1989; Lewis and Glennerster 1996; Lewis 2004). The difference, however, is that care giving to older relatives who are frail and/or suffering from chronic illness often represents an increase in care that surpasses the bounds of normal or usual care in the family. For example, here is a quote from a service user during care needs assessment:

My two daughters have been sharing it amongst themselves to look after me since I had my stroke. This is because of the love we have for one another. Am used to seeing them or their children and we can relate to one another without difficulty.

Care giving to older relatives because of reduced functional abilities involves a significant amount of time and energy over extended periods. It involves tasks that may be unpleasant and uncomfortable, which are likely to be non-reciprocal, and it is often a role that had not been anticipated by the caregiver (Tessler and Gamache 2000). When these unanticipated roles are incongruent with stereotypical gender expectations, for example when a male caregiver must attend to an older relative's bathing or laundry, the stress can be exacerbated. Although much of the empirical research on care giving limits the definition of family caregivers to blood relatives, factors such as the family, nationality, race/ethnicity, and the sexual orientation of the ill relative may dictate broader conceptualisations. These may include a more extended kin and non-kin relationship (Barusch 1995; Tessler and Gamache 2000).

Extent of Family Care Giving
The expectation and prevalence of care giving in families is high (Carers National Association 1996, 2001; Help the Aged 2002). As social welfare costs rise, there are increasing obligations placed on family members, primarily females, to undertake care giving responsibilities (Olson 1994; Barusch 1995). One might argue that a caregiver is needed for every person with health-related mobility and self-care limitations that make it difficult to take care of personal needs such as dressing, bathing, and moving around the home (Carers National Association 2001; Twigg 2006). Indeed, a recent national survey of caregivers reported that there were 7.5 million households which met the broad criteria for the presence of a caregiver in the previous twelve months. Of course, not all older relatives who need assistance from family caregivers actually receive this help and this may happen for a variety of reasons, including a lack of family

23

members or unwillingness or inability of family members to provide care (Machin and Waldfogel 1994; Qureshi et al 2002, Carvel 2007).

The provision of care by family members to other family members who become dependent due to old age and or physical disabilities is not a new phenomenon. Families have always provided care to their dependent family members. However, there is now growing recognition among service providers and researchers that family care giving will become more significant in the future because of the shortage of formal social care workers, demographic change, socio-economic dimensions, and social changes in the 21st century that are anticipated to continue into the next century (World Bank 1994; United Nations Organisation 1999, 2002; King's Fund 2006). Family care giving is seen to be natural and nurturing to accommodate all family members for example, a family caregiver expressed her views as follows:

> I feel happy looking after them, because they're my parents... and I look after them, as well as my sisters. I don't like to see them struggle. I support them emotionally really. I see them every week, usually speak to them on the phone once or twice a week and strangers cannot assume this responsibility.

A number of trends are likely to shape the future of informal care giving. Life expectancy and the ageing of the population have increased dramatically during the last hundred years with the world's population ageing at a fast rate, especially in developed countries. A shift in the epidemiology of disease from acute to chronic diseases and a decrease in accidental deaths in developed countries have resulted in an increase in the number of people with functional activity and mobility limitations (Organisation for Economic Cooperation and Development 1998; Lefley 2001; UN 2002). The number of multigenerational families has increased, resulting in a growing number of older caregivers as well as increased numbers in the "sandwich generation" which has produced reconstituted families such as stepmother/father, stepsons/daughters and half sisters/ brothers.

Most families within these groups combine their efforts to provide care for older relatives to whom they have no biological link at all (Delaney and Delaney 2003). With greater numbers of women (the traditional caregivers) in the labour market, the combination of working outside the home and providing care for dependent family members has become increasingly more difficult (Pickard et al 2000; Lowe 2003). Increased geographic mobility in England and the movement of youth from rural to urban areas in search of employment has distanced adult children from older relatives and siblings (Barusch 1995; Lewis 2006). Here is a quote from a service user during care needs assessment:

> It's always an advantage I suppose because then you feel you're being cared for by people who care rather than people who are just paid for it. Your family would not rush you about because of the love that exists... you know.

Nature of Family Care Giving

The roles and functions of family caregivers vary by the type and stage of the illness, frailty and disability, and include both direct and indirect activities. Direct activities can include provision of personal care tasks (helping to get washed, bathing, getting dressed and toileting), and health care tasks (catheter care, assistance with medication), as well as checking and monitoring tasks such as continuous supervision and telephone monitoring to ensure the health and safety of older relatives. Indirect tasks include care management (such as locating services, co-ordinating service use, monitoring services, or advocacy), household tasks (such as cooking, cleaning, shopping, and financial management) and transporting family members to medical appointments and day care programmes (Noelker and Bass 1994; Carers and Disabled Children Act - DoH 2000). Family care giving to some extent an instinct that is unavoidable and a family caregiver summarised her feelings as follows:

> Oh it's obviously concerning and worrying... I mean we trundle along together; we don't do much because he doesn't want to do anything, and he'd rather sleep all day if he had his choice... I made sure his care is provided the way he would have done it himself. You cannot trust strangers because you don't know them and some of them cannot be relied upon.

The intensity with which some or all of these care giving activities are performed varies widely. Some caregivers have only limited types of involvement for a few hours a week whereas other caregivers might provide more than forty hours a week of care and be on call twenty-four hours per day (Wistow et al 2002a; Hasler 2000; Sales and Leason 2004). There are, for example, significant differences in care giving responsibilities and tasks for caregivers of older spouses or older siblings as compared to caregivers of cared for persons with mental illness, with the former involving more hands-on care. In other words, personal care and household chores potentially carry social stigma and pervasive worry about the relative's safety (Twigg and Atkin 1994; Quershi et al 2002). Family care giving and care needs assessment for older relatives are interrelated and the boundary between them is insignificant during care giving. Therefore, family caregivers undertaking the care needs assessment and providing care would promote holistic functional activities of daily living to the older relatives in their own home.

Reliability and Consistency

In this context, family directed care system is a shift toward a new paradigm within the wider welfare systems. The service framework would enhance social care delivery and diversity that contributes to wider choices and flexibility within the social care market. This book is intended to highlight the need for pluralistic economy of social care and this would be above the micro-level of social care delivery available to older people in general. The care pathway would help in policy reconstruction that could narrow the limitations and gaps on political ideologies, and current legislation such as the NHS and Community Care Act (DoH 1990) and Carers and Disabled Children Act (DoH 2000). The care model would form part of modernisation of social care services that is aimed to diversify the social care market and choices and control amongst the services users.

The conceptual service framework would have a deliberate strategy to preserve core family values; tradition, culture and purpose, at the same time stimulate, encourage progress, and change within the wider welfare service. The family is a social structure; their values provide the opportunity to respect the co-operative strength of culturally accepted decision-making process relevant to long-term care for older people (Roberts 1995; Lewis 2002, 2006). Yet, inconsistent political ideologies and limitations within legislation and policies, have contributed to dependency culture amongst the users of public services (Gordon 1988; Wilkinson 1999, 2000). Family norms and values are unique and transferable between cultural settings. It could be argued that there is no similar motivational coherence in the complex of cultures and disparate family structures, which must be served by the state (Young and Willmott 1957; Phillipson et al 2001). This view is supported by a comment from a service user:

> I went away... in May and I never come back until the mid July because I went to stay with my other daughter in Wales, and then to my sister, because they are my family and that is how my daughter wants my care to be provided...Some families have a set of rules and values that guides all family members. These values may be shared and observed between generations, this is how my family have been.

The characteristics of the family directed support care systems include: early intervention; targeted support where families understand the aims of services to enhance wellbeing; support which uses and builds on strengths which tackles the main problems and vulnerabilities; and a whole family approach. This considers how services and plans should fit together rather than considering problems in isolation. According to Twigg and Altkin (1994) and Phillipson et al (2001), family care system could usefully be employed to the early consideration of care and applied to strategic recovering plans, which emerge from the family interactions and shared initiatives. The care model would assist in the reconnection and reconstruction of care needs assessment and safety parameters with support plans, for which the family members can understand, and produced by themselves. They would when appropriate source external help to bridge gaps within the family care systems and to support them in their caring role (Rosser and Harris 1965; McRae 1999; Breda et al 2006).

Family involvement is aimed to promote active partnership – a three-dimensional approach – the family, the older relative and the state. Partnerships in this context implies a measure of quality and agreed decision sharing between the stakeholders on how best to plan and manage the growing older people's population and their care needs (Finch 1995). In almost all the adult social care services such as older people service where the professionals, the family members and service users are sometimes involved in assessment, there are usually both stark and subtle differences in authority, responsibility and influence between them (Walker 1998; Lymbery 1998a, 2004; Postle 2002). Differences of opinion could lead to waiting list for assessment and care, complaints against social services and poor quality of care that, if not resolved might lead to abusive situation in the long-run. In practice most users would welcome shared responsibilities between the family and social services. A service user described her views as follows:

> Well, I think they've got to share the care package and pay regular visits and I think that would be a lot for families with young children to bear. I think sharing the care package will definitely reduce pressure on the family caregivers... They have their own lives and family commitments other than caring for their older relatives.

In policy framework, working in partnership with the families is an aspiration to share knowledge, responsibilities and to maximise resources for the benefit of all stakeholders. The concept of partnership with and within families is conditional, layered and would sometimes be completely elusive. However, the service framework could be a measure to elevate personal social services beyond professional dominated care system to deliberate and practical engagement. Family members tend to respond to situations where they have been involved from the beginning, and their views are listened to and respected. Linking with long-term care planning for older relatives, family participants would respond constructively if they are being asked what they would recommend, and what plans and services they believe would benefit their older relatives (Finch 1989, 1995; Wellman and Wortley 1989; Bauld et al 2000; Qureshi et al 2002).

Culture and Traditional Philosophy

Family participation in designing functional activates of daily living of an older relatives is aimed to be a care pathway and a robust set of idea that is continually challenged and refined as we move forward with preparedness to changing policies, procedures and structures in the wider welfare systems. It is systematic approach to reinvent traditional family care systems and the opportunities inherited within that system, so that key support and interfaces are maintained. The family would remain relevant and responsive to the growing population and care needs of older people (Evandrous et al 2001). The key emphasis of this framework is to broaden the stakeholders' views about the potential of traditional family care systems that has the abilities to design and deliver personalised social care to their older relatives. The model would maintain a high level of quality and human capacity consistent to meet the increasing older relative's aspirations (Murray et al 1999; Lewis 2004 & 2006). Reflecting on practice based-knowledge and experience, a service user illustrated her views as follows:

> As a parent, you brought your children up and you assisted them with all their needs and make sure they are all right... don't you? There's nothing wrong for them to assist you when you're older and unable to do simple things. In return you expect them to do the same for you; I feel it is a duty... I see nothing wrong with that.

The focal point on traditional family care systems as a progressive care system for the future would reassert for example, two things: Firstly, family is socially reliable and trusted than strangers as some would see family care giving as a duty. Secondly, family is seen as the basis for stability and strong moral foundations in society, albeit alongside a recognition that the family is changing (reconstituted and composite family) (Finch and Mason 1993; Wilkinson 1998, 2000; Lewis 2006). In this book, a traditional family oriented care system could offer stability and security in a fast moving world of globalisation, migration, demographic change and smaller family units. Giddens (1998, 2001) argued that the family should be seen as part of that world, expressing flexibility and inclusive to form a long lasting contemporary welfare systems.

According to Blair (1998a), the decline in traditional family care systems has contributed to a greater welfare dependency, especially among older people. Blair argues that the reassertion of strong collective values in the community requires the family. The family has a lot to offer particularly that associated with personal social services for older relatives and the growing welfare dependency. Yet, inconsistent political ideologies and political rhetoric has not kept pace with increasing socio-economic needs of family caregivers in order that they would continue in their caring role. According to Wilkinson (1998), she argues that:

> There has been an unhealthy polarisation between liberals who affirm individualism, and tend to take a relativistic view of family values and structures, and conservatives who talk a lot about values but neglect household economies. The result of this is a policy impasse. Yet we have been presented with a false choice. Problems being experienced by families today are rooted both in economic stress and in family disintegration. Any progressive family policy must address both these issues or it will fail (1998).

Allen and Perkins (1995) vividly demonstrated that family is unique because the family both requires and underpins individual responsibilities in promoting family holistic wellbeing for example, continuing care for older relatives and children. Similarly, Finch and Mason (1993), Conekin and Di (1999) and Glendinning et al (2002) argued that the state alone would not be able to meet the increasing needs of older people in the future, unless families are involved in reshaping the power balance. Chapter four below discusses the need for family members to undertake older relative's care needs assessment and care giving for payment.

Welfare State and Changes within the Family Units

A further difficulty with social policy is that it is broad based and ignores changes to other areas within the welfare system, in particular that relating to older people and their families (Townsend 1983; Phillipson et al 1986; Glennerster 2006). One extension of the social policy conflict idea might be that just as older people are failing to moderate claims at the micro-level of the welfare system, they are also exerting undue pressure at the macro-level of the family. According to this school of thought, and numerous reports and research, such as Harris (1998) and the Carers National Association (2001) documentary on the plight of carers, might be one indication of the way in which older people have continued to receive a disproportionate share, not only of state support, but also of that arising from family care giving of different kinds (King's Fund 2006). Ogawa and Rutherford (1997) and Grundy 1991 and 2000) have shown that older people are altering the claims made on other family members due to changing family structure such as the reconstituted family unit.

The dominant sociological view for a number of years has been that, as Shanas (1976 and 79) argued, that older people turn first to their families for help, then to neighbours and finally to the state because they expect their families to help in case of need. Wenger (1984), demonstrated that most care comes from the family and that most people thought that this was where the responsibility should lie. This view has been central to the philosophy of community care both in the UK and elsewhere (Glaser et al 1998; Glendinning et al 2002). However, it can be argued that there is no consistent evidence to support this perspective. Indeed, research is now available which suggests that care preferences are changing (Whitley 1981; Carvel 2007). This reflects an important shift in the relationship between older people and their families. The argument is that there is a readjustment in attitudes towards receiving, and to a lesser extent giving care. The implication is that the hidden welfare service is shrinking in part because some family caregivers are ageing, especially women whose age ranged between 45 and 80 (Lowe 2003; Carvel 2006 and 2007).

A key point about care preference is a public opinion survey, which shows the extent to which adults of all ages focus on the state rather than the family in respect of needs for financial, health and social care support (Salvage et al 1989; Phillipson 1990; Glennester 2006). A Gallup survey carried out in the 1980s and 1990s found that older people believe responsibilities for their care should "shift towards the state" (Carvel 2007). The survey found that most people believed that the state should take primary responsibility for the provision of older people's care and that this was financially affordable. Although there was support for the idea of help being means-tested, people were reluctant to use available means to fund their own care. Walker (1995) explored views about care-dependent groups and the relationship between the state, professional groups and informal carers. He concluded that despite the fact that the public may not be pleased with the policy such as Caring for People (Department of Health and Social Security 1989); they were unwilling to shift a burden of care onto their family carers, which in practice meant an increasing burden for women in particular.

However, surveys of public opinion in 1996 and 2007 found that most people who were not currently carers expected their family or friends would look after them if they could no longer look after themselves (Carers National Association 1996 and Carvel 2007). The greatest burden was seen to fall upon the family. More than six out of ten of non-carers believed that the state should pay the major share of the cost of care, 45% feeling that central government and 17% that the local authority should pay the major cost, while 28% felt that the cost should be shared evenly between the family and the state. A very small proportion (less than 5%) believed that the cost of this should fall primarily upon the cared for person and their family (Carers National Association 1996).

Family care giving in the 2000s and beyond, although still present and stronger in some social groups and cultures than others, presents an opportunity to address the growing population of older people and their demand for care. However, low childbirth rates among the present generation might be a dilemma for reciprocal family care giving (Evandrous and Falkingham 1998; Phillipson et al 2001). This perception could likely be altered in terms of the conditions under which care is provided and the range of care tasks that can be offered to older relatives in the community. Economic migration of family members and the lifestyle of family caregivers as well as their economic wellbeing are all factors that need to be taken into account in future family care giving. According to Wistow et al (2002a&b) and the Commission for Social Care Inspectorate's (2007) assertions, older people might be re-assessing the kind of demand they can make within the family. This is because family units have changed from what it was during the original studies by Townsend (1957).

Conclusion

The exploration of the ideological positions of this book and conceptual policy framework has highlighted wide ranging strengths and opportunities that families and traditional family care systems could occupy in a modernised welfare service. These have the hallmark of social re-engineering and behavioural change within the family and the wider society to rethink new dimensions to continuing care for older relatives now and the future. The chapter has also provided an opportunity for the policy makers to re-examine the conventional service frameworks and reformulate appropriate measures to accommodate family care system as a core service framework. This book has therefore advocated for reconsideration and re-interpretation of social policy for older people as time is no long in the hands of the politicians to delay any further. The growing older people population is now a time bomb that could explode at any time.

Chapter Three:
The Need for and Potential of Family Care Management Involving Payment for Family Assessment and Care Giving

Introduction

This chapter considers the unique position of traditional family care systems and the functions of the family caregivers to undertake care needs assessment and provide care for older relatives for payment. This is the main focus of the chapter. This care model is known as "family-directed support systems". The chapter is sub-divided into five sections: Care needs assessment and personalisation of care; personalisation of services and care management approach; eligibility criteria and care management, advantages of personalisation and family care systems and supporting relationships between the stakeholders. Each of the sub-themes will be examined, highlighting some of the relevant issues that are linked with traditional family care giving and the chapter will draw on references from previous studies relevant to social policy for older people.

Care Needs Assessment and Personalisation of Services

A needs assessment is a process of establishing the needs of a service user. It may trigger a package of services that would help to sustain the life and activities of the daily living of a cared for person (NHS and Community Care Act 1990). The assessment may be carried out at various stages, so it could serve several goals, and it falls into three main types: 1) **Assessment for eligibility for services** and funding for someone who is not yet using services. 2) A s**imple needs assessment** to establish the most appropriate care plan, care pathway and package of care for a client to determine the diversity of their needs, if they are not too complex. 3) A **comprehensive needs assessment** help establish a full care plan for a client with complex needs, but also to evaluate the appropriateness of the service provided and to determine whether it is necessary to add, withdraw or in other ways make changes to the service packages (DoH 1990 - NHS and Community Care Act; Milner and O'Byrne 2002; DoH 2002f).

The first option is an eligibility assessment, which is the least resource consuming of the three and may be the initial step in a care episode (Hughes 1995; Lymbery 2001 & 2004a). If the client's needs are not too complex, the second option – a simple needs assessment – could be added to the eligibility process. For example, if an older relative needs help with cooking or laundry, and there is no family or friends available, the decision to provide meal services or washing services will not need a full needs assessment. The third option of a full evaluation is more costly but is needed in integrated care for people with complex needs to organise, provide and manage their care by different agencies or professionals.

Objectives and Intended Outcomes of Needs Assessment

The overall objective of the needs assessment is to obtain a picture of the client's needs that balances their requests for services with an objective analysis of their needs in the light of limited public funding and spending decisions (Lymbery 2001 & 2004a). This process involves ethical decisions, drawing on concepts such as equity, integrity, and autonomy. The needs assessment is intended to support family members or social workers in planning care for service users and to ensure that service developments are matched to the greatest needs as possible and to priorities between different. Depending on the reason for the needs assessment as outlined in the previous section, objectives that are more direct can be identified.

Simple Needs Assessment

A simple needs assessment may be performed to suggest a care plan delivery for people with few needs where only a few service packages will be considered. In some cases, this simple approach is adequate (Kendall et al 2003; DoH 2002). For example, when only a few services are considered, such as shopping, cooking or transport services, a simple needs assessment will enable service providers to find out whether the client is satisfied with the quality, and to detect whether a rearrangement is necessary. It can also enable management to make sure their services are producing the desired results. This assessment can also enable screening into more complex care.

Comprehensive Needs Assessment

Where clients have critical and substantial needs, professionals and informal carers are presented with more challenges. Here the needs assessment provides a structure for collecting the information from all parties involved, where this "global" information is used for all as a basis for visualising the needs for integration of services and shared responsibilities. Comprehensive needs assessment is carried out to establish support plans, care package that could sustain the cared for persons' holistic functional activities of daily living. Such an integrated package would facilitate an opportunity for choice and control through which quality of care could be delivered. Thus, support plan is subject for reviews in order to evaluate outcomes, such as resource consumption and caregiver's stresses (Phillip, Ray and Ogg 2003a & b; Lowe 2003; King's Fund 2006).

The purpose of needs assessment is to obtain a view of the client's needs that is fuller than that of the eligibility assessment. The reason for this is that a broader assessment might highlight new needs that have not been dealt with earlier. At first glimpse, this may lead to higher resource consumption, but, according to Payne (2000) and Lloyd (2002), identifying and handling needs earlier on improves the quality of care and quality of life. It also enables social workers to priorities their activities better. A needs assessment at this level provides a reliable summary description of the area or agency workload to request and allocate resources more appropriately. Social workers can use this information to help intertwine the services that are provided by formal and family caregivers in the care of the older person. This information also enables care provider agencies to meet their legal requirements to provide social services with information about their work (Challis and Hughes 2002). A comprehensive social care assessment embraces:

Key Guides for Social Care Assessment Process and Practice

The assessment generally involves finding out the background information about a service users and their carers:

- *Biographical details*: The following information is required: name, age, marital status, religion, and so on.

- *Self-perceived needs:* The assessment should always start with the views of the individual and his/her wishes.

- *Self-care*: What the person can do for him/herself, such as washing, cooking, dressing, etc.An important point here is that the potential of the person should also be taken into account. For example, an older widower may have been used to being looked after by his wife.When assessed, he makes little effort to do anything for himself.The care manager must decide what the appropriate level of help for him, given his own capacities and the resources available.

- *Physical health*:This is crucial, and a proper assessment of the person's health will be undertaken by a health professional, most probably the G.P.Health problems often require both medical and social services, as ill health may prevent a person from performing self-care adequately.

- *Mental health*: An assessment by an appropriate health professional is required, probably the community psychiatrist. The mental health of the individual may effect his/her perception of needs and the ability to perform a number of routine daily activities.

- *Use of medicines*: Many people need regular medication, and a common problem is the inability to self-administer this.Problems resulting from inadequate medication may affect the broader lifestyle of the person and their ability to achieve an adequate standard of self-care.

- *Abilities, attitude and lifestyle*: Each person is unique in their views, abilities, lifestyle and personal range of family and friends upon whom they can rely.The assessment must take this into account and must not simply stereotype an individual, for example as an older person with arthritis living alone.

- *Race and culture*:The assessment must include an awareness of race and cultural wishes that spring from this.The impact of racism on people's lives should also be considered.

- *Personal history*:Any relevant information that the individual provides which may help to understand their present needs, for example, the death of a partner, or past involvement with health or social services which they regard as unsatisfactory and which affects their attitude to the current assessment, should be taken into account.

- *Carer Needs*:These have been more formally addressed by legislation.Where there is currently someone providing care, his or her views also need to be taken into account.The individual being assessed, and the care manage, may make false assumptions about the wishes and attitudes of the carer. Both Carers

(Recognition and Services) Act 1995 and the Carers and Disabled Children Act 2000 has provided yardstick to the needs of carers and their qualification for assessment and care in their own right. Thus carers' needs should be covered in an assessment, taking into consideration of the following:

- Relationship to the individual being assessed (for example, spouses or daughter)
- Care provided (cooking and shopping)
- expressed needs for support
- Wishes and preferences
- Nature of the relationship (warm/distant).

- *Financial assessment:* The financial assessment looks at the person's income and savings in order to see how much, if anything, the person has to pay for services.The local authority has traditionally decided its own rules for domiciliary, day and short term (respite) care, for permanent care in residential/nursing home they must follow nationally laid down rules.

NHS Continuing Health Care and NHS Funded Nursing Care

The NHS continuing healthcare is the name given to a package of care which is arranged and funded solely by the NHS for individual outside of hospital who has ongoing healthcare needs. Continuing healthcare can be provided in any setting, including in the community (in the clients' own home) or a care home. NHS continuing healthcare is free, unlike help from social services for which a financial charge may be made depending on your income and savings. If clients own his/her own home, this means that the NHS will pay for healthcare and personal care. If healthcare is provided a care home, the NHS also pays for the client's care home fees, including board and accommodation. Anyone assessed as having a certain level of care needs may receive NHS continuing healthcare. It is not dependent on a particular disease, diagnosis or condition, or who provides the care, or where that care is provided. If the clients' overall care needs show that his/her primary need is a health need, the client should be eligible for NHS continuing healthcare, his/hercare will be funded by the NHS, but this is subject to review, and should his/her care needs change the funding arrangements may also change.

Whether someone has a primary health need is assessed by looking at all of their care needs and relating them to four indicators:

- **Nature**: this describes the characteristics and type of the individuals' needs and the overall effect these needs have on the individual, including the type of interventions required to manage those needs.

- **Complexity:** this about how the individual's needs present and interact, the level of skill required to monitor the symptoms, treat the condition and, or manage the care.

- **Intensity:** this is about the extent and severity of the individual's needs and the support needed to meet them, which includes the need for sustained/ongoing care.

- **Unpredictability:** this is about how hard it is to predict changes in an individual's needs that might create challenges in managing them, including the risk to the individual's health if adequate and timely care is not provided.

How Decision for Eligibility is made

The whole of the decision making process should be person centred. This means putting the individual and their views about their needs and the care and support required at the centre of the process. It also means making sure that the individual plays a full role in the assessment and decision making process and gets support to do this where needed. This could be by the individual asking a friend or relative to help them explain their views. Primary care trusts (PCTs) should also make the individual aware of advocacy support services that may be able to assist. An approach to the primary Care trust (PCT) to consider continuing NHS health care should be made in any case where the older person has complex health care needs. Once a determination has been made, the service needs do not meet the criteria for continuing health care an "Registered Nursing Care Contribution" (RNCC) assessment should be completed (DH 2007). Where a determination is for NHS funded continuing health care, the PCT for the geographical area in which the older person resides is responsible for the full cost of funding. The older person can access NHS continuing Health Care in a nursing or mental disorder unit. If the service user was placed after 1 April 2006, the placing PCT remains responsible for providing the continuing care as directed by the National Health Service (Functions of Strategic Health Authorities and PCT Administrative Arrangements (England) (Amendment) Regulations 2007).

After the 12 weeks review, if it is deemed that the situation has stabilised, the PCT funding will cease in consultation with social services authority through the support planning process following a joint review between health and social services. Good practice demonstrates that the 12 weeks review should be joint health and social care. Until transfer of funding is agreed, primary care trust will continue to be financially responsible for nursing care. However, where the withdrawal of PCT funding is contested by relatives or service users, it remains also the PCT funding responsibility until resolution is accorded by all concerned (DH 2007). Directly linked with the NHS continuing care funding, it should be noted that longevity and complex medical conditions such as organic cognitive impairment has led to the enactment and introduction of Mental Capacity Act (2005). The Act has influenced social work skill, assessment and practice giving social workers delegated power to carry out Mental Capacity Assessment with any potential service user who is deemed incapable to make informed decisions regarding to his/her long-tern care needs and management.

Mental Capacity Act (2005)

The Act provides a statutory framework to empower and protect vulnerable people who are not able to make their own decisions. It makes it clear who can make decisions, which situations, and how they should go about this. It enables people to plan ahead for a time when they lose capacity. The Act is underpinned by a set of five key principles stated in section 1 of the Act: 1) A presumption of capacity - every adult has the right to make his/her own decisions and must be assumed to have capacity to do so unless it is proved otherwise. 2) The right for individual to be supported to make their own decisions – people must be given all appropriate help before anyone concludes that they cannot make their own decisions. 3) That the individual must retain the right to make what might be seen as eccentric or unwise decisions. 4) Best interest – anything done for or on behalf of people without capacity must be in their own best interest.

Mental Capacity Assessment empowers social workers or allied professionals to undertake capacity assessment in order to Safeguarding Vulnerable People under certain conditions. The Act deals with two situations where a designated decision – maker can act on behalf of someone who lacks capacity: 1) Lasting powers of attorney; the Act allows a person to appoint an attorney to act on their behalf if they should lose capacity in the future. This is like the current Enduring Power of Attorney, but the Act also allows people to let an attorney make health and welfare decisions. 2) Court appointed deputies – the Act provides for a system of court appointed deputies to replace the current system of receivership in the Court of Protection. Deputies will be able to make decision on welfare, healthcare and financial matters are authorise by the Court but will not be able to refuse consent to life – sustaining treatment. They will only be appointed if the Court cannot make a one-off decision to resolve the issue. 3) Independent Mental Capacity Advocate (IMCA) an IMCA is someone appointed to support a person who lacks capacity but has no one to speak for them. The IMCA makes representations about the person's wishes, feelings, beliefs and values at the same time as bringing to the attention of the decision – maker all factors that are relevant to the decision. The IMCA can challenge the decision-maker on behalf of the person lacking capacity if necessary.

Deprivation of Liberty

Deprivation of Liberty - Section 6 of Mental Capacity Act (2005) defines restraint as the use or threat of force where an incapacitated person resists, and any restriction of liberty or movement whether or not the person resists. Restraint is only permitted if the person using it reasonably believes it is necessary to prevent harm to the incapacitated person, and if the restraint used is proportionate to the likelihood and seriousness of the harm. Section 6(5) makes it clear that an act depriving a person of his or her liberty within the meaning of article 5(1) of the European Convention on Human Rights cannot be an act to which section 5 provides any protection (MCA 2005).

Implications for Social Workers

The Mental Capacity Act will require major changes across health and social services to enable its requirements to be implemented. To make these changes, decision will be required at both strategic management and operational levels.Equally the Act will change significantly the way in which capacity is assessed i.e. capacity to make particular decisions rather than capacity to make any decision. These changes will allow others in addition to psychiatrists to make these decisions. As a result of this it is probable that there will be differences in opinion between psychiatrists who may have undertaken a critical assessment of capacity and social workers who may have made an assessment on a social model. Where local negotiation fails the only other means of resolution is legal challenges through the courts. To avoid this scenario it is imperative that a local protocol is put in place to discuss these areas of cases and where the necessary arbitrate between the two parties.

Enabling Individual Older People to Control their Care

Needs which falls outside the critical or substantial criteria will not be met by social services authority. However, within support planning, in meeting a critical or substantial need, an individual older person may also meet moderate or low needs as a bi-product within their preferred care options (DH 2002). The local authority is obliged to balance the needs of its service users with its financial responsibilities to the tax payer. Different benchmarks will clearly arise for different service users and risk groups, alongside some care packages/services having elements of "front loading" so that, over time, older people are supported to be increasingly independent and support can be expected to reduce. Generally, the opportunity for older people to have their social care needs met at home extends to the point where the cost of doing so is less than or equal to the cost of meeting their needs via provision of an alternative appropriate service. Setting best value cost ceilings is good practice, but Fair Access to Carer Services guidance (DH 2002) states; "if spending above the ceiling can make a different to an individual, then the local authority should consider doing so".

Personalisation and Care Management Approach

A needs assessment may be carried out as part of an evaluation of the services given. If this is a standardised and comprehensive procedure, this could solve various problems such as stress and isolation in the community (DoH 1990 - NHS and Community Care Act). The existing services may not meet the client's needs for a number of reasons. For example, if they are based on historical factors, they may be obsolete or out of line with the client's current needs. Without re-assessment of needs and services, historical inequalities or errors may be perpetuated (Bauld et al 2000; Lymbery and Millward 2001). Another possibility is that the services may be too demand-led. In this case, only those who ask for the services receive them, and only the most urgent needs are met. This prevents service users from obtaining early information about the client's physical, cognitive or social decline that may enable them to put preventative measures in place (Lymbery 1998a; Postle 2002).

Another problem is that needs that are obvious at a first glance may not always be the ones to address first (Commission for Social Care Inspectorate 2006c). Risks such as malnutrition, isolation and exclusion are more easily prevented if service providers carry out a more structured needs assessment based on full knowledge of the service user's needs and declining functions with increasing age. For example, if a client is suffering from incontinence, a simple solution would be for the family to source incontinence pads rather than making a thorough investigation of the cause of the incontinence. This risk is evident if the family believes incontinence is a natural part of being old – as with reduced appetite or thirst – and these misconceptions can be a hotbed for ageism and stereotypic views of older people (Bauld et al 2000; Qureshi et al 2002). But by requesting a more thorough picture of the client's needs and analysing the educational needs of the family/user, the providers can clarify which problems are simply due to ageing and which require treatment. In some cases, this may also enable preventative treatment in certain conditions if they are discovered sufficiently early.

Assessment Outcomes

Needs assessment would not resolve all issues. It may even give rise to new questions such as; how does one deal with a situation where there is a conflict between client needs and client demands and preferences? How should one link present service activities to the needs assessment? How can one include risk management to the assessment process? To deal with a discrepancy between client needs and preferences, it is important to involve the client and their relatives in the care planning process. This situation should also be dealt within team discussions to ensure a true balance between the key stakeholders. With detailed information of the client's needs, we can more easily priorities and remodel different services, if we consider them based on eligible criteria matrix (Postle 2002; Carey 2003). Furthermore, if the assessment is carried out comprehensively, this increases the likelihood of discovering risk areas and preventing risks such as violence or abuse between spouses, and environmental risks such as lack of heating. Thus, good assessment has the potential to yield holistic information that could be used to minimise social care needs plummeting to critical and substantial needs in the long term. It could also reduce costs of care giving (Lloyd 2002; Phillip, Ray and Ogg 2003).

Eligibility Criteria and Care Management Process

The care model would be family led rather than professional led. The rationale is that family members, who have lived alongside and have known the older relatives probably throughout their lives, will have a better understanding of their holistic functional activities of daily living than a social care worker may have. It is family led because many older people might have chronic illness or an organic ailment such as dementia or chronic obstructive pulmonary disease (Chronic Obstructive Pulmonary Disease) that could impede their ability to carry out their activities of daily living. The model advances the opportunity for the family to carry out holistic care needs assessment of their older relatives and provide care for payment. The model would only be available for those families who wish to access and participate in the care pathway. The family's involvement is aimed at reducing waiting lists for assessment and care on the one hand and on the other hand to reduce the pressure upon the formal care workers to attend to the needs of older people as demanded by legislation.

The need to address some of the current and future care needs for older people presents serious human and ethical dilemmas for social services and the family (Royal Commission on Long-Term Care for Older People 1999; Commission Social Care Inspectorate 2006d). This means that for the last three decades the political discourse and changes have been about individual rights and choices to live and receive care in the community (Lloyd 2002; Lymbery 2004a). Perhaps in the 21st century, it is therefore important that we remember families' inter-dependence. Under the NHS and Community Care Act (DoH 1990) local authorities have a duty to provide information to users and potential users of community care. This includes receiving referrals for assessment for social care needs and provision of community care as deemed appropriate.

Within this care model, all referrals for assessment and care giving would be made to social services directly to the screening department that filters referrals. In line with the existing practice pertaining either to direct provision or direct payments, the screening care worker would discuss the availability of the care models such as direct payments and direct provision with the referrer to help choose a care pathway. Depending on the choice of care model, the social care screening worker would forward the appropriate referral to the local team manager for a decision and then contact the referrer or family member to start the assessment and care processes (National Health Service and Community Care Act DoH 1990).

During referral to social services, if the referrer or family member wishes to access the family care pathway, a meeting or series of meetings would be scheduled between the family and a social worker to consider the options in more detail. This would provide the opportunity to discuss the care model, the processes and possible difficulties that might arise during care giving, and how to address potential problems without a breakdown in care. The social worker would give advice on assessment processes, the type of forms needed for completion, monitoring and training on the use of specialist equipment such as a hoist, care provision and ways of reporting or responding to incidents during care giving. At the end of the process, the family care assessor or the caregiver would be well informed about assessment of care needs, the content of a care plan and provision of care in line with that plan. The detailed information provided to the family would form part of their learning curve as well as the understanding, knowledge and skills appropriate to pursue family care.

To proceed with the care model, the social worker would send the assessment and care plan forms to the potential family assessor or caregiver to be completed and returned to the local team manager for consideration and action. The dedicated worker would liaise with the potential user or their family to acknowledge receipt of the completed forms and provide advice and information about funding the care package, contracts, the service users' financial contribution towards care provision, payment to the caregiver and implementation of the care model. The social worker, through the team manager, would present the case and care plan to the care planning board to be considered for funding and validation of the care option. The dedicated worker and the user or their family would be advised of the decision of the care planning board. The dedicated worker would therefore be tasked to guide the family and ensure that all processes and procedures relevant to the family care model are adhered to.

The dedicated worker would be known as the family care advisor with whom the family would always relate to for advice on carer's breaks, review of the care packages or difficulties with payment and benefits. This collaborative work would be a continuous process until stability of care giving was achieved. The worker would also be a link to the multi-disciplinary team and would forward all relevant documents such as finance and contracts to all relevant departments or teams within the service in order to ratify the care model. The worker would be responsible for updating the social services information systems for easy access and retrieval of information as and when appropriate within the services. At the end of the assessment and implementation of the care pathway, the case would be closed to the dedicated worker or team and would be banked with the review team for yearly review unless the family requested an interim review because of unforeseen circumstances in the family (Milner and O'Byrne 2002).

The care model has some similarities with the family group conferencing and kinship care perspectives in children's and family services but differs in application and process. With the family-directed support care model, the family member would carry out the assessment of needs and draw up the care plan in consultation with the cared for person, whereas with family group case conferencing a qualified social worker carries out the assessment of needs and determines the care plan in advance. The objectives of the model are to enable older relatives to exert their rights and choices of where and who they wish to have as a caregiver, either in their own home or in a residential care home (Milner and O'Byrne 2002).

The focus is on ensuring that the family makes all key decisions in consultation with the older relative (if they have capacity) and provides care if they wish for payment. This is in contrast with present system where the social worker assesses the needs and decides who provides care to the service user. Nonetheless, if disagreement arose between the family and their social worker during the assessment and care process, the matter would be referred to the operational team manager who would try to resolve the problem. However, if the problem persisted, the family would be offered the opportunity to make a formal complaint through the county council's complaints department, which would follow the due process of complaints procedures. The model would not be a process of queue jumping, but the ability of users and their families to exercise their rights under the Human Rights Act (1998 ss 5, 8, and 10). It is also about the enhancement of hospital discharges and prevention of unnecessary hospital admission (DoH 2000 & 2003; Lymbery and Butler 2004) and the promotion of the National Service Framework for older people (DoH 2001a).

Critical Social Work Practice and Family Care Giving

The care model would form a working partnership between the family, the older relatives and the dedicated worker and social services. This is so that the family would not feel that the care for their older relative had been "dumped on" them. The dedicated worker would monitor the care package in alliance with the family caregiver and this agreement would form part of the family care plan.

The levels of monitoring would depend upon the nature of care package in place and complexity of needs. Usually the initial 4-6 weeks review would be undertaken by the caseworker who would act upon the outcome of the review and inform all the stakeholders with full documentation (National Health Service and Community Care Act - DoH 1990). From the initiation of the care model, the worker would clearly advise the family or the user about the monitoring arrangements, as well as professional responsibilities to facilitate the care pathway.

Of paramount importance to the care model is the issue of clarity of information and processes. The family caregivers would need to understand the eligibility matrix of assessment and care as well as boundaries between care giving and payment to them. This would help them to make choices in comparison with the existing service frameworks of direct payments and direct provision. A high degree of clear information about the model from the beginning would be useful for the family caregivers, as this would help them to overcome any concerns about the model. The information pack would also include details of relevant support systems from other agencies such as housing, health, and the Department for Work and Pensions (DWP). The worker would assist the users and their families to access these services as and when necessary. The service framework is not intended to be an isolated service but would form part of the core services framework within social services.

Family directed support care systems model would promote intergenerational participation in family care giving. It is in family groups that we learn how to be members of society and how to behave in different settings. Once learnt, this pattern of co-existence and support is difficult to forget (Burgess 1960; Lewis 2004). Family influence remains strong throughout the rest of our lives. We need to remember that the family structure in England and other developed countries is changing (Office of Population Census and Survey (1995 and 96); Office for National Statistics 2001). Essentially, there are more single persons and single households with no families to take on the care model. The care needs of this group would still be addressed by the social services as at present. Nevertheless, the proposed family-directed support care systems have some perceived advantages and disadvantages like the conventional care models of direct provision and direct payments.

Benefits of Personalisation and Family Care Systems

Although the literature on family care giving tends to highlight the negative effects of caregivers' roles, numerous studies have investigated the positive impact of tending to an older relative's care needs. Findings from a Swedish study, for example, suggest that satisfaction from care giving derives from varied sources and that most caregivers do experience some kind of benefit (Lundh 1999). Some families of adults with chronic illness report instrumental as well as psychological reward, notably when the care recipient is able to reciprocate with emotional contributions to the family. Elderly spousal caregivers of persons with organic and chronic disease studied in a cross-national study were found to derive satisfaction from doing their job well, experiencing affection and companionship from the care recipient, and fulfilling a perceived dutiful role (Murray et al 1999; Lewis 2004 & 2006).

Consequently, the care model has the potential to preserve the stability of care giving by the family, to respect the views and opinion of the users and their families, to help them feel safe from potential abuse, to maintain links with the family, siblings and friends, to sustain their racial and cultural heritage, and to remain within their own community (Delaney and Delaney 2003). The care model would be proactive, reducing waiting time for assessment and care and enhancing the psychosocial wellbeing of the service user and their family. On the other hand, it would shift responsibility away from the state towards the family, making them accountable as well as giving them the ownership of assessment and care of older relatives. It would also develop specialisms within the adult and social care service within social services and the wider welfare systems. The care pathway has the potential to reduce pressure on care workers as well as complaints from families and users about poor quality of care giving (Noelker and Bass 1994; Wistow et al 2002).

As stated previously, family directed support care giving can have positive effects for the caregiver as well the user (Bulger, Wandersman and Goldman 1993; Beach et al. 2000). For example, Beach and his co-authors found that elderly spousal caregivers demonstrated improved mental and physical health as care giving activity increased. Adult children who are caregivers to elderly parents report that they find care giving gratifying because they can pay back the care that their parents provided to them when they were young. In addition, caregivers report that being a caregiver helps them gain inner strength or learn new skills.

Family intervention intends to provide families and family caregivers with social and psychological support, and in most instances information about a particular chronic illness, as well as suggestions for coping with that illness. Support for the family would be professionally led, ensuring that the family was well informed about the support systems available and that their needs were met to avoid care breakdown. It might also be family led, given their understanding of the older relative's care needs, likes and dislike during care giving. The former is often conducted in hospitals and community care settings, whereas the latter typically takes place in community meeting places such as family homes, churches or social care centres (Bulger et al 1993; Delaney and Delaney 2003).

Psycho-educational interventions have, as a principal component, a focus on changing family coping behaviours and attitudes. In addition to the presentation of information, they typically include skills training for families in communication and problem solving. Although the designated target of change is the family, the ultimate impact of psycho-education is on the patient's symptoms and functioning. Psycho-educational interventions are provided in both multi-family and single family formats and are most likely to be found in culturally sensitive ethnic communities (Young et al 1999; Phillipson et al 2001).

Family involvement in assessment and care for older relatives could in part help older people achieve their wish to be cared for by the people they know and who are committed to assist them with their care needs in their own home (Lewis 2004). According to the Carers National Association (2001), paid family care giving would be cost effective for social services, because payment to family caregivers above the minimum wage would still be less than the declared rates paid to independent provider agencies. The opportunity to access the market would give families and users the choice to explore and evaluate what is available in times of potential pressures and crisis in the family. It would also offer the opportunity to have a break and rebuild their efforts to continue care giving roles for their older relatives. Interaction between elements in the market would foster continuity of care giving, carers' breaks and quality assurance during care giving. It would give social services the opportunity to plan, develop and commission care packages that could cope with the aspirations of older people in the 21st century and beyond (Wistow et al 2002). Allowing the current frameworks to run their course within the welfare services means there would be a significant reduction in care and support services for both older people and their families. The inclusion of families and social networks would add a new dimension that could facilitate a flexible care market within the wider welfare system).

The family-directed support care model would mean recognising the importance of the economic wellbeing of the family caregivers which in turn could revive the family's' involvement in care giving to older relatives. Given the present economic situation, any family policy that neglects the economic wellbeing of the caregivers could repress the enthusiasm of many family caregivers to commit their time and skills for their older relatives' care (Hughes et al 1999; Qureshi and Walker 1998; King's Fund 2006). Present legislation, such as the NHS and Community Care Act (DoH 1990) and Community Care (Direct Payments) Act (DoH 1996a) and Carers and Disabled Children Act (DoH 2000), focuses on two main frameworks of direct provision and direct payments, arguably restricting the potential of the social welfare market to meet the increasing demand for care by older people (Royal Commission on Long Term Care for Older People 1999). At present, despite the recommendations of the NHS and Community Care Act (DoH 1990), social services are failing to fully engage family caregivers and social networks such as friends, neighbours and voluntary sector organisations as partners in responding to the shortages of both social workers and carers. In view of the inflexibility in the social care market, the proposed social care model could rejuvenate the market.

Family-directed support care systems would lead to greater emphasis on quality of care giving, a person-centred approach, education and the learning process between the stakeholders. The model could also strengthen the economic dimensions of care provision through expanding demand and supply, choices; service availability and accessibility of the social care market. Social services would be in a stronger position to commission care for older relatives through their family caregivers, as well as enabling them to plan and access the social care market of their choice. This approach would synchronise with the aspirations of the growing population of older people who wish their care to be provided in their own home and in the community they know (Hasler 2000; Wanless 2006).

The care model could also be a source of income generation for family caregivers and their nuclear or reconstituted families. Extra income earned might improve their lifestyle and standard of living, giving them economic power that could enhance their health and psychosocial wellbeing during care giving. Payment to them would be taxable and would be a source of income to both national and local government. This might to some extent elevate some family caregivers above poverty levels, and give them job satisfaction as well as acquiring skills they could utilise in the social care market at the end of care giving to older relatives.

The needs assessment would help families to obtain a view of the client's needs that is fuller than that of the eligibility assessment (DoH 2002b). The reason for this is that a broader assessment might highlight new needs that had not been dealt with earlier. At first glance, this might lead to higher resource consumption, but evidence shows that identifying and handling needs earlier on improves the quality of care and quality of life. It also enables family caregivers to prioritise their activities better within the family (Milner and O'Byrne 2002; Payne 2000). For the manager of the social work team, a needs assessment at this level would provide a reliable summary description of the area or agency workload in order to request and allocate resources more appropriately. Managers could use this information to help intertwine the services that are delivered by several participants in the care of the older person. This information could also enable providers to meet their legal reporting requirements (Bauld et al 2000).

For the older relative, the needs assessment would be the means by which they are seen as an individual and could interact with the family caregiver and the social services, and could discuss and influence the care provided (Lymbery 2001; DoH 2001a - National Service Framework for Older People). For the manager, the needs assessment would be a more objective tool with which he or she could balance the resource availability. On a systemic level, the needs assessment would provide information that enabled social services to scrutinise the costs of care compared to other costs in society, and to determine priorities. It can be tempting to make a rough estimate of what a client might need, but it pays off to try and obtain a more holistic view that may include functional deficiencies that need to be supported by various services. This would strengthen the bases for further rehabilitation to support the service user and their family caregivers (Lymbery 1998a, 2000). A holistic view of this kind could enable data to be gathered through one process to be used for all levels of decision making from the care given via management of staff and resources to national monitoring.

Supporting Relationships between the Stakeholders

Family care systems and personalisation of services illuminates the future of adult and older people's services and the potential of family care giving to revitalise and strengthen the social care market within the wider welfare system. By applying family theory on the basis of present and past knowledge, we would be able to learn and form a strategic partnership with the family with a view to responding proactively in the social market. Family theory in this instance has the potential to educate and provide the necessary stimulus to react to the increasing demand for care now and in the future. Even if the consequences of the mixed economy of social care now and in the future have been correctly predicted, it would still be necessary to shape and re-shape these forces in accordance with explicit views about what constitutes desirable outcomes. Changing demography means political and economic analysis is needed in order to redesign and deliver a person-centred approach to older relatives through their family members for payment (Royal Commission on Long-Term on Care for Older People 1999; Evandrous et al 2001; O'Hara 2004).

The model raises the question of choice and what constitutes desirable directions and destinations. In other words, it requires at least a minimal framework of principles and purposes to guide not only the consistent development of policy and practice, but also to provide a reference point for scrutiny, review and revision. Means and Smith (1995 and 1998a) and Walker (1984) advance the principle of empowerment through users' involvement and provide a useful example of why such frameworks and processes are necessary. While user engagement and empowerment have undoubtedly become more fully developed over the last twenty years in social care, there is also much evidence to demonstrate that they are not rooted in everyday routines and practices in services for older people and their families (Glennerster 2006).

Accommodating family-directed support care systems for payment would strengthen what Alcock (1998) called local governance, which has three benefits: inclusiveness as opposed to exclusion enhanced social network, and redefinition of the older people's agenda. These factors would help older relatives to come to terms with their care needs. It is a contemporary expression of Seebohm's (Donnison 1968) development agenda for the community as a whole system, where family members would be fully involved in their older relatives care. It also represents community characteristics fundamental to enabling the personal fulfilment of wellbeing of the individual and the groups for whom social care has special responsibilities. Social services would concentrate on commissioning and enabling services within the wider welfare services for older people and other vulnerable users of services in the community (Wistow et al 2002).

Public opinion supported by previous studies such Phillipson et al (2001), Wistow et al (2002a) and Lewis and Meredith (1988), Wilkinson (1998, 2000) and Lewis (2006), advance the uniqueness of family care giving which represents a desired outcome of social care for older relatives, both in terms of the general role in the building of community capacity and also the contribution of that capacity to the lifestyles of those who are over 65 years old, with particular needs and requirements. The approach advocates that older relatives, families, social networks and whole community roles are fully interdependent in terms of realising each of the three categories of the outcomes in meeting the needs of older people in their own home. One of the strengths of the care model is that it places greater emphasis on developing a holistic perspective on family care giving to meet the needs of adult and older relatives for payment, a move towards securing their own economic wellbeing, promoting community involvement and provision of services in the older relatives' own home.

Conclusion

In view of the wider ramifications of the growing older people population and their care needs as well as the constriction of the formal social care workers, this chapter has justified the need for family's involvements to partake in the cared for persons care needs assessment and care for payment. The chapter has highlighted a number of advantages of the model and compared and contrasted them with the existing care pathways. The joint ownership, family control and choice of care approach have been found to give an important boost to the lives of older people and their families. It could be argued that this model of care has some similarities with the direct payments scheme, but the difference is that because of the age, mental capacity, medical conditions, frailty and disabilities of some older people they may not be as capable as even adults with disabilities to take control and make decisions about their care. To offer older people the best possible social care, it could be argued that joint decision making with their families is essential. In addition to the potential of family care giving, this chapter has identified that the model would be cost effective in comparison with the existing service frameworks of direct payment and direct provision. However, the book also identified some challenges that could deflect the care model for example, economic migration of some families and burden on families.

Chapter Four (A):
The Service Users' Views

Introduction

The aims of this chapter are to highlight the views of the service users about the care model. The results of the study are narrated under each of the key themes and categories that emerged from the interview data. The findings represent what the users wanted from their families and their experience within the welfare system. Their views demonstrated a unique understanding of family-directed support care systems.

Part One of this chapter begins by analysing the family care giving and that concentrates on two themes: emotional needs and practical tasks are seen as important to the service users during care giving. The third and fourth part discusses the issues around reservations about the proposed care model and resistance to family care needs assessment and care giving for payment. The fifth and the sixth sub-sections include analytical dimensions of enabling support systems and socio-economic factors that could influence decision-making on family care in the long term.

The participants were able to reflect from both a vignette and their own life experiences to answer the research questions and these provided broader and wide-ranging data for the study. Reflecting on these themes, the analysis adopted the common phrases used by the service users during the interviews to describe their experiences. These phrases were used to frame the categories for in-depth analysis of the data.

The study revealed two important dimensions that are pertinent to family care giving: the emotional dimension and the practical tasks of care giving. The elements are analysed separately and the objectives for dividing the theme into two are to identify the essence of emotional wellbeing and why service users want their families to provide care for them rather than strangers.

Emotional Dimensions

Emotional themes represent some of the psychosocial values that are unique to a person and can only be understood by that person or those around that person within their own environment. Emotional care for some older relatives helps sometimes to promote a speedy recovery and psychosocial wellbeing during care giving. Some participants said that family care giving would assure them that people they know and who share their background and history could meet their needs. They would see a face they knew and that person would understand their needs. It would give them the opportunity to share family problems and difficulties.

Most of them said they like to hold on to things they cherish and admire, and they are not willing to lose that family relationship whilst they can remember the values and history attached to it. The study revealed that about two-third of the group (11/15) preferred to receive care from their family members. In contrast, a significant minority (4/15) disagreed with the majority's views (see resistance to family involvement below). The Thematic Dimension One below gives a graphic illustration of why some older relatives preferred to receive care from their family.

Thematic Dimension 1

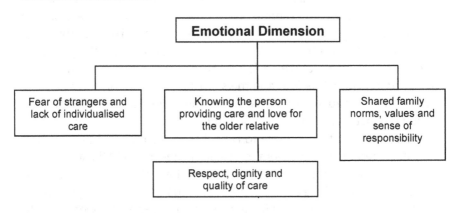

Fear of Strangers and lack of individualised care

The majority of this group (11/15) said that they saw many faces visiting them for care giving, and therefore they didn't know who their main caregivers were and this raises their anxiety and worries. They believed that the caregivers didn't understand their character either, and as a result they would be exposing themselves and their entire household to vulnerability. Care provision in most cases was inconsistent, lacking individualised care and quality because they saw different carers most of the time. They linked mistrust and fear of strangers to the extent that some stated they might not be safe in the hands of strangers or that those strangers would not be able to assist them adequately with their holistic care needs. Some highlighted their individuality; therefore they need their individualised care to be promoted at all times. These situations could have some negative impact in the way older people perceive care giving from strangers.

You like to know who you are bringing into your house. You've got to be careful these days who you are bringing in, or taking on. You read stories in the newspapers where people take things that are not theirs and so you wouldn't just employ anyone would you? (SU2).

You see different carers all the time and some lack the basic knowledge of your individualised care and you have to explain yourself all the time while they rush you about. This is worrying you know...I will prefer my family to care for me (SU7).

Knowing the Person Providing Care and Love for Older Relative

The majority of the service users (14) thought that knowing the person providing care would make them feel more relaxed (e.g. SU1, 2, 5) and enable them to partake in their care giving process. Knowing the caregiver has some psychological advantages and this could help to avoid misunderstanding and possible care breakdown. A number of the service users (e.g.SU1, 6, 10) said that having a family caregiver assisting them meant that they didn't have to see different faces but instead only saw faces of people who recognised and understood their needs. Care giving is correlated with the love you have for the older relative and most thought that there is enduring love within the family that binds them together, otherwise family caregivers would not devote their time for care giving.

Anyhow, they are your family and they know your ways. Our girls they used to be carers... home help and then they are trained into that, but there you are, that's how it goes, you know them and what they can offer and you don't have to explain yourself to them (SU5).

It's always an advantage I suppose because then you feel you're being cared for by people who care rather than people who are just paid for it. Your family would not rush you about because of the love that exists... you know (SU6).

Shared Family Norms, Values and Sense of Responsibility

Care giving is intertwined with shared family acumen and the family's way of life, which is understood by all family members (SU 2, 3, 6, 14). Most group members said that their family knew them well and could support their customs and traditions better than strangers. Some believed that they would prefer to have their family members to assist them because strangers lack the knowledge of their family history and could be ambivalent towards older people (e.g. SU 10, 12). Some thought that family care giving is a responsibility that has been reciprocated from one generation to another. Strangers would rather rush about and go their way and some may even have no concerns about older people's welfare.

> I went away... in May and I never come back until the mid July because I went to stay with my other daughter in Wales, and then to my sister, because they are my family and that is how my daughter wants my care to be provided...Some families have a set of rules and values that guides all family members. These values may be shared and observed between generations, this is how my family have been (SU3).

> Depends on the family background, I think some family members would take their time to look after their older parents without rushing them about and John and Maggie is an example isn't it... (SU10)

> I think some strangers can be erratic in their approach and could be ambivalent towards older people and their plight; this is why I prefer my family (SU12.

Respect, Dignity and Quality of Care

Almost all the group members (14/15) indicated the need for carers to observe respect and dignity whilst offering quality care to users. Care giving encompasses identifying care needs deficit, negotiating, and establishing a pathway to accomplish that (e.g. SU3, 4, 6, 9 and 14). This paves the way for compromise and developing a caring relationship that would be beneficial to all without risk of care breakdown. Some expressed that care encompasses giving and receiving respect from one another and this potentially forms part of the family norms and values, which are accorded to older relatives. This view reflects the behaviour in some families, which strangers would not tolerate during care giving (e.g. SU4 and 14). Some of the participants stated despite their older relative's behaviour towards them, the family would still have to accommodate it. Some thought that not all strangers would accept such behaviours or attitude from the cared for person (e.g. SU3, 6). Some extracts from the vignette provide an illustration:

I can be difficult some time and lash out to my daughter and grandchildren simply because am unable to do simple things that am used to do. My daughter does bear with me because she knows how I feel and she understands my condition. I don't think strangers would take it lightly with me when am rude to them, but my daughter can take it... I think this could be applicable to John and Maggie (SU4).

My kids drive me up the wall but as you get older you get more cantankerous, men especially... the men I do know. Anyhow, they are your family; they know you and respect that attitude and behaviour, I suppose this may be relevant to John and Maggie his daughter (SU14).

Practical Tasks during Care Giving

There is a conceptual link between emotional wellbeing and practical tasks (e.g. feeling, guilt, duty) during care giving. This is why some of the research participants said they would prefer to receive care from their family. Over three-quarters of this group stated that their families were able to assist them with their holistic care needs (e.g. housework, personal hygiene, meals preparation). A few number of the participants felt otherwise (see resistance to family involvement below). However, over two third (11/15) believed that care giving involved contacts with the cared for person and practical aspects were an essential part of care giving. The study showed that care giving includes continuous assessment and evaluation of needs in order to identify changing needs such as: personal hygiene needs meals preparation, shopping, and laundry which the older relatives expressed as essential components of their functional activities of daily living. The Thematic Dimension Two below reveals the categories under which the family caregivers would support older relatives with their needs.

Thematic Dimension 2

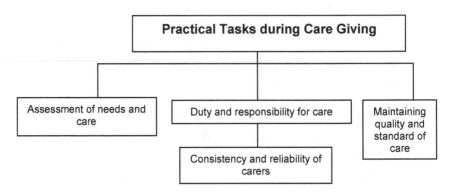

Assessment of Needs and Care

The study showed that a large number (9/15) of the service users thought they would be in control when their family caregivers were assessing their care needs and providing care for them. This is because their family members understood their likes and dislikes, as they had known them for most of their lives (e.g. S.U 1, 7, 9). Most of them said that their family caregivers could tell them the best way to meet and manage their care needs tasks within the household, while social care staff might not have an in-depth understanding of their needs and how they have coped. Some acknowledged that assessment of needs and care giving can sometimes be complex and unpleasant but they preferred their family to undertake that role on board (e.g. SU 2, 4, 12). The shared view was that their family would take their time and ensure that emotional and practical tasks were accommodated during care giving, whereas this might not be possible with social workers. Although they understood the significance of families' involvement in assessment and care, some (4/15) thought that social workers were qualified to carry out their assessment of needs. Another two participants stated that assessment should be a joint approach between their family and social workers (e.g. SU 5).

> I mean there is not a lot for me to worry about. Oh, she does practically everything, and I can't see any more point in saying... I think I will feel more confident for her to assess and care for me as she has been doing (SU1).

> My daughter does my laundry, meals, personal care... everything you know she is my family... I feel she will be able to assess my needs better than a social worker because she knows me and my care needs (SU7).

You have to go closer to the woods to see the trees... I think it will take social workers more time to understand my needs. I think my family knows me better and are more suitable to assess my care needs and provide care for me. That is my opinion... (SU12).

Duty and Responsibility for Care

Duty of care duty responsibility was mentioned by a large number of service users to demonstrate their feeling of what family care giving is all about (SU1, 5, 14, and 15). Some stated that their family members were duty bound to assist them with their care needs. Responsibility went beyond ad-hoc or emergency care giving and some participants reaffirmed that it is an engagement, which involves holistic activities of daily living which strangers would not have the time to provide (e.g. SU 6, 12). For some participants, duty and responsibility involved undertaking practical and psychosocial tasks in order to continue to support them in achieving their aspirations. In contrast, a significant minority (4/15) did not share the views expressed by the majority (see both resistance and reservations about family care giving below). These vignette response extracts provide an illustration:

As a parent, you brought your children up and you assisted them with all their needs and make sure they are all right... don't you? There's nothing wrong for them to assist you when you're older and unable to do simple things. In return you expect them to do the same for you; I feel it is a duty... I see nothing wrong why Maggie can't help John (SU6).

Maggie's presence will help John to possibly live longer, don't forget he lost his wife and Maggie has been there to support and they share responsibilities together (SU9).

Maintaining Quality and Standards of Care

Some of the group members talked about maintaining quality care standards and tidiness that they were used to in their own home and felt that an unkempt household would upset them and their relatives. This shows the significance of maintaining standards that people are used to and would like to adhere to. People are individuals and what one person appreciates may not be applicable to another, a consistent level of standards was identified as a major issue for some older people during care (e.g. SU3, 7, 13). Most of them expressed such a view although social services do not offer general housework for older people to meet their hygiene needs which are paramount during care giving. Their family caregivers would not mind helping them maintain a clean environment that would be conducive to them and their caregivers (e.g. SU 3, 11, 15).

> I have always lived on my own since my husband died and my children married and gone. I have always kept my little home clean and tidy and I want it to remain the same and my daughter-in-law has helped me to keep it that way. I don't think strangers would.... No I like tidiness (SU1).

> I like my house to be clean and tidy always, although social services do not offer help with that...but my family knows the standard I am used to... I like it that way; you know... strangers don't understand you... (SU3).

Consistency and Reliability of Carers

An interesting finding was that family caregivers were perceived to be more consistent and reliable than strangers (SU1, 7, 15). Some inter-depended on their family caregiver as they share their care needs to get by the day; this means that care giving is consistent and reliable. Even when the family caregiver is not living under the same roof, the majority of the group members (12/15) said that they knew when their family caregiver would visit them. They could spend more time with them and assist them to the best of their abilities. Some (e.g. SU1, 5, 10) revealed that family members would not disappoint them with their care needs and that the support offered and the presence of family made them feels relieved. Most thought that it would make them feel relaxed knowing that help was at hand, and if family carers were unable to arrive at the expected time they would inform them of alternative arrangements to be made (e.g. SU8, 13). The reliability of the family caregivers helped to promote psychosocial health and wellbeing as they knew that they would be assisted with their care needs.

> Yes, because we are all in a family you see, we are a very close family. We depend on one another to get by... If my daughter-in-law can't do it, one of her boys will do it, or if I want anything, they will come over and help me (SU1).

> I mean, we've always been a good family, we've always worked well together... you get families that don't want to know their parents. I am lucky ...and I know that, and I appreciate that but then I did look after my children and I did everything I could for them (SU 8).

It goes round and round, yes they will be there for me otherwise, they will make alternative arrangements... (SU15).

Resistance to Family Involvement

The study findings showed that about a quarter of the service users (4/15) would not like their family members to participate in their care giving. They said that family structure had changed because of marriage and migration of their family members to different parts of the country for economic reasons. Most pointed out that distance and sensitive nature of personal care giving could create a barrier for family care giving. A few argued that family care giving would mean that the older relatives had to interfere with the lives of their family members and that might increase pressure on them and their nuclear family. Some maintained that their resistance did not mean they were totally against family reciprocity, but only that they wished to remain as independent of their family as possible and be supported by social services. Thematic Dimension Three demonstrates some of the views expressed by some users who disagreed the philosophy of the proposed care model.

Thematic Dimension 3

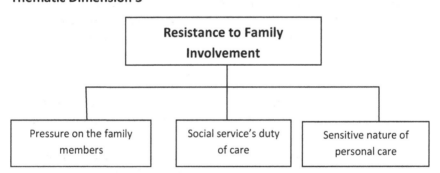

Pressure on the Family Members

The study revealed that some participants believed that care giving was very demanding and involving, and they stated that such pressures and commitments could compromise family relationships. They preferred to receive care from social services rather than from their family members. Some argued that increasing demand on their family might be counter-productive because of the pressure they had to bear by trying to assist them. This could aggravate family conflicts. For some family conflict could be avoided by not involving their family for example:

I have my two daughters, they live locally with their own families, and I can't every time call them out to help me. They lead busy lives and bringing up their own children, I don't think it is fair on them and that could break up their marriage because of pressure on them. I don't want to take that blame (SU3).

My family is there for me if I need them, but not for caring for me. No I have my care from social services. Caring can be very demanding and involving and these would increase pressure on them, coupled with their other activities. If I need them, I will let them know... (SU12).

Social Services' Duty of Care

About a quarter of this group (e.g. SU10, 11 and 13) argued that social services had a duty to provide care to them without family involvement. Some stated that they had paid their National Insurance contributions and taxes during the time they were in employment and these supposedly should fund their care needs from cradle to grave. They argued that it was not the role of their family to take over the responsibilities that should be fulfilled by the state.

I'm from the older generation and since the war we have paid our stamps in full and we were promised care from cradle to grave and why can't social services provide care to us now...? It is their duty and not the family's and when you're old nobody wants you ... No that is not good. I prefer social people you know it's their duty (SU12).

Social services have a duty as I am aware of to look after people like John and myself, though I am still fairly independent, but I have only one visit from social service a day to help me with my wash. They should send someone to help John as Maggie has her own life. Care giving is very demanding and can increase pressure on Maggie, resulting in conflict... (SU13).

Sensitive Nature of Personal Care

A significant minority of the participants (4/15) stated that some older people tried to avoid asking their families for assistance and only did so when other avenues had been exhausted. Families were seen as the last resort when it came to care giving. Some professed that care giving was a very personal matter and a sensitive issue and that they would not accept assistance from their families. They argued that personal care giving would change family relationships and roles, as they would feel ashamed and embarrassed for their siblings to offer personal care. This can be a very depressing and degrading moment for some family members:

> Care giving is personal and private and why social services can't provide care to older people. Families can only help that's my opinion but not taking over what social services are supposed to do, why not... I can't have my son to give me a wash; it's not fair on both of us ...that is very private... no...no (SU11).

> I prefer to have social services to care for me and not my family more over to offer personal care... no it is very personal and involving. There are certain things that you will not want your family to help you with... (SU12).

Enabling Support Systems

Back-up support systems were mentioned by all the participants even those that were not in support of the care model (15/15). Some stated the reasons why they thought their caregivers should be supported in their caring role. The common view was that aids and equipment, shared care packages, respite and day care would contribute immensely to the achievement of their aspiration to be cared for at home by their relatives. Most believed that family-directed support care systems were about sharing responsibilities amongst family members and social services. With this understanding, families would not relinquish their efforts and wait for social services for help during care giving. A number thought that this perspective was dependent on the family's shared wisdom, values and their belief systems and hence some families would always rally round to support their older relatives at all costs. On the other hand, some families might not be supportive of their older relatives; therefore, care reciprocity is not unique to all families. Service users knows what they want and would be obliged to receive some support from both their family and social services in order to remain in their own home for as long as possible. Thematic Dimension Four below represents three key support systems that service users thought would help them attend their holistic functional care needs in the community:

Thematic Dimension 4

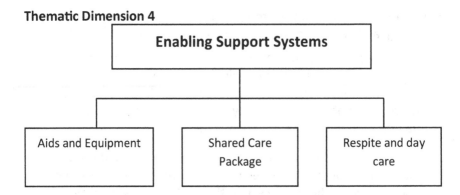

Enabling Support Systems

Aids and Equipment | Shared Care Package | Respite and day care

Aids and Equipment

Most participants drew a link between aids, equipment, and interdependence with their caregivers (e.g. SU3, 8, 11, 13). Some saw aids and equipment as enabling support systems that would help the family caregivers or the formal caregivers to manage their care needs well. Most revealed how desperately they needed equipment to enhance independence. Some gave examples of how equipment had helped them regain some form of independence and mobility (e.g. SU1, 6, 9, and 11). Most of them disclosed how equipment had assisted them to manage, reduce risks of falls in their own home and maintain their health and safety, whilst they continued to be interdependent with their family (e.g. SU2 and 3). All of the participants (15/15) thought that aids and equipment were essential for them and their family caregivers:

> I think ...if I fall over... I've got this... I'm attached to a telephone ...they say to me, are you all right, and if not, they send somebody out to me, which is a good thing. At least you know that somebody is somewhere monitoring you in the house. I think that is the main advantage (SU2).

> I've got a walking frame and I get about walking like that but I've got to have a bag to put on it to carry things in and out and my daughter, she goes to work from about 9 a.m. until about 4 p.m., see... five days a week, she works for herself, so I've got the access to the front room (SU3).

Shared Care Package

A large number of the participants for example SU2, 7, 9, and 15 to mention the few, indicated that their family members did not have adequate time for their care. Some expressed that care giving was very challenging and they stressed the need for shared care packages with social services. A number of them believed this option would relieve stresses and pressures that were likely to affect decision making about care giving and commitment. The majority (11/15) highlighted the need for collaboration between the family and social services and was hopeful this would enhance carers' breaks. Some suggested that shared care packages should include the provision of personal care, shopping and laundry. These support services would go a long way towards assisting their caregivers.

Well, I think they've got to share the care package and pay regular visits and I think that would be a lot for families with young children to bear. I think sharing the care package will definitely reduce pressure on the family caregivers... They have their own lives and family commitments other than caring for their older relatives (SU5).

I don't really see that there's a lot more one could do. The support for the carers is the main thing and I can't see that you can do much more than make sure they are washed and dressed and fed, and be comfortable. Well, I mean it is about collaboration with social services and share the burden... (SU6).

This is where the social people could help Maggie by attending her, off hand, not for any direct treatment, but twice a week, so that Maggie has got someone to look forward to, to come in and think, well I won't worry, I'll have so and so to help me...see what I mean (SU15).

Respite and Day Care

Almost all the group members (11/15) expressed the frustration and helplessness of being together with their caregiver day in and day out and demanding assistance with care. Most thought that some of the family caregivers were over burdened and stressed because of combining care giving and their own activities of daily living (e.g. SU 3, 8, 15). Multitasking of this nature could lead to ill feeling between them and the only way to address these potential difficulties was by offering them frequent respite or day care. The study also found that some of the service users were isolated in their own homes and that they had no family members or neighbours around to socialise with them. For some this could be very frustrating and sometimes depressing (e.g. SU 6, 10, 14). The common view was that day and respite care would be an opportunity for them to remain in their own home for as long as possible. These vignette extracts below provide an illustration:

> I mean being together all the time could lead to ill feelings and potential abuse due to constant demand for care. I think day care and rolling respite would help to reduce tension between John and Maggie (SU3).

> Well, I suppose in the first place, Maggie would be under a lot of pressure caring for her father and going to work. The social service should help her by offering carers' breaks, offering John the chance to attend day centre or respite care from time to time (SU6).

Socio-economic Dimensions

A large number of the group (8/15) thought that their families had their own financial needs and lifestyle they had to meet during care giving, and as a result they should be paid. Many of them (e.g. SU4, 7, 8, 13) said, since care giving to older relatives could be time consuming and challenging for some family members, they might not have the time to pursue and achieve their own socio-economic goals. However, a significant minority (4/15) were of the opinion that family caregivers should not get paid for care giving to their older relatives. Some argued that family care giving was about paying back and expressing love for their older relatives. Some felt that it was immoral to pay family members for care giving. A few (3/15) were undecided and acknowledged the advantages and disadvantages of paying family members for care giving. The study uncovered a divergence of views amongst older relatives regarding payment to their family caregivers. Some of their views are represented in Thematic Dimension Five below.

Thematic Dimension 5

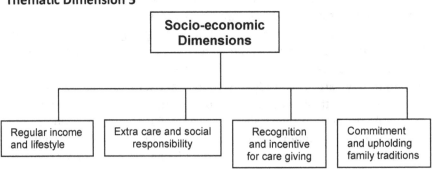

Regular Income and Lifestyle

The study showed that the majority (8/15) of the group thought that their caregivers should be paid by the state in order to maintain the lifestyle and standard of living they were used to (mortgage, holidays, rent, council tax and car ownership). Some argued that payment would help their family caregivers plan for their future and address those needs. Most argued that families' socio-economic circumstances could be more complicated than offering care to their older relatives (e.g. SU2, 8, 5, and 14) and supported the view that family caregivers should be paid.

> I think Maggie should be paid for caring for John; otherwise, social service will have to pay anyone coming to help him... Maggie has her own life and has expenses to run, despite the fact that she lives with her father (SU8).

> If they've had to give a job up, with a younger family I would say yes, but if it's an older family, if she's working for a pension, that's her future, therefore...a younger person, it would pay you to pay them to keep them at home, but depending how much... they have lifestyle to maintain (SU14).

However, some (4/15) did not share the majority view, but they contended that family care giving was about love, paying back and keeping in line with family norms and values. Payment to family caregivers would erode those belief systems. Love for older relatives and care giving could not be measured in monetary terms. Therefore, payment to family caregivers would not be acceptable. A few (3/15) participants were undecided, but state that they would prefer their family members to assist them with their care needs.

> I for one do not agree with payment to family members caring for their older relatives, what is family for...? Caring is about love and sort of paying back, no it is immoral... (SU1).

> I don't think that families should be paid...to me caring for older relatives is about keeping in line with family norms and values, payment to family caregivers would erode those belief systems. John and Maggie are probably without payment... (SU12).

Extra Care and Social Responsibility

A significant number of the group members (8/15) reported that their families needed a regular income of some sort in order to sustain their socio-economic circumstances. In some families, money paid to family caregivers could be used to buy extra care to support their social responsibilities, which they would not otherwise afford without extra income. Some argued that maintaining social responsibilities and meeting constant demand for care without extra income could jeopardise continuing care for the entire family systems (e.g. SU2, 3, 5 and 8).Some service users assisted their family caregivers with their financial needs but that support was not enough to supplement their earnings from employment or business to uphold their commitment for care. Most explained that payment to their caregivers was money well spent and this would help to raise them above poverty level. The caregivers knew that any amount of time they spent for caring was remunerated. For some payment was a form of social responsibility to encourage the caregivers to carry on care giving, irrespective of their physical and psychological strains (e.g. SU5, 9, 13).

> Well, it is because she is tied... the only other thing that the money would be useful for is to have someone in now and again to sit in with John, so that she can go out, say have a night out or an afternoon out shopping, and if he can't be left alone then someone to sit in, but nobody will do it for nothing (SU1).

> No, that's not fair. Well, she's got the boys growing up hasn't she, and all their things cost money, and one's like, well one is leaving school next year, and the other one has got a year or so, and everything costs money doesn't it... it's not right that she should keep me free... no, it isn't. Extra income into the family would help her support the boys and this will ease off financial difficulties that might otherwise make her not to continue helping me (SU3).

In contrast, some (7/15) questioned the contribution the income earned during care giving would make to some families; although this depended on the family's earning power and socio-economic class (e.g. SU7, 11). Almost one half rejected payment to family caregivers and cautioned that it could disrupt family cohesion, their social network and their belief systems (e.g. SU6, 13). According to this view, the family should be self-reliant without seeking to be paid by the state. Others thought that what was important within the family was seeing themselves as a unit without a division and treating each and every one of them as a "tangible asset" that promoted family reciprocity.

Although family circumstances differ, I don't think that payment to family carers would make much difference in some families. I strongly oppose that... (SU13).

I am against payment to family caregivers, as this could disrupt family cohesion and social network. A united family can be a tangible asset that promotes family care system... (SU6).

Recognition and Incentive for Care Giving

Some of the service users said that payment could be seen as an incentive to attract and retain family members who would not have otherwise have thought of assisting older relatives with their care needs (e.g. SU2, 5, 9, and 15). Most (11/15) recognised that care giving was a difficult task and they acknowledged the time and efforts their family caregivers invested in them. The tendency is that family caregivers would provide quality care than strangers would otherwise. A number of them argued that family care giving would help them achieve stability and this approach would help relieve anxiety and fear. Most contended that not many families could do without an income and some argued that payment to family caregivers would draw them closer to take part in care giving (e.g. SU2, 5, 8, and 14).

Caring for older relatives is not a job for many family members. I think paying family members I hope will act as incentive and could attract those who would not have dream of caring for older relatives (SU9).

I think payment to family members caring for their older relatives would be, a sort of recognition, for their time and commitment. This in my view shows that social service recognise family commitment and reward them...you know (SU11).

About a quarter of the participants (4/15) rebuffed the concept of recognition and incentive, and argued that reciprocal family care giving was about promoting intergenerational heritage which could bind the family together (SU3, 7). Payment was not a remedy to attract family members to participate in care giving. What was necessary was the love of caring for older relatives as part of family history (SU13). For them, care giving was an instinct that grew with them and was passed on to the next generation.

For me financial compensation to family caregivers is an inappropriate way of recruiting caregivers to meet the increasing

69

demand for care from older people. Family care giving is about upholding and preserving that part of history that makes the family unique and binding (SU6).

I mean caring is an instinct that grows within you and that is passed on between generations. Love is immeasurable and does not tarnish but evolves with time. I am against payment to families... (SU13).

Commitment and Upholding Family Traditions

Service users did not expect their families to care for them for nothing. They understood the economic difficulties many families face these days in achieving their potential. Almost all the participants (12/15) professed that payment was not a new phenomenon and sometimes family caregivers were paid in kind (gifts, holidays). Some were paid in cash, for example paying grandchildren's school fees or a monthly or weekly allowance for their upkeep. Some argued that such payment in this context would formalise a tradition that has been in existence for many years (e.g. SU 2, 5, 12). The only difference emanating from the study was that any payment to the family caregivers would be made by social services. Family caregivers would be committed hence; they know they would be paid for their services. Most thought that many older relatives would continue to offer financial assistance to their family caregivers as a gesture of goodwill and continuing parental support to their siblings (e.g. SU 6, 8, 14).

I would have liked my son to be paid for the support and care he gives to me. Any little income would help and when that money is paid, it remains in the family rather than being paid to a stranger... you know you should think of your family first... and support them financially if you are in that position (SU5).

Reservations about Family Care Giving

Although a large number of the group (11/15) wished to receive care from their family, yet a significant number (7/15) expressed some reservations about family-directed support care systems because of constraints upon the family caregiver such as meeting the needs of their nuclear family as well as their older relatives. Most thought that family caregivers would be pressurised to a certain degree during care giving. Some of them indicated that, there might be some circumstance within the family that would be beyond the control of the family caregivers. Some argued that situations of this nature might interrupt care giving and potentially put them and their caregiver at risk. Family care giving might represent an opportunity to balance the power of care responsibilities between the state and the family. However, the implementation of the care model might present some dilemmas to all the key stakeholders. Thematic Dimension Six below illustrate some of their views:

Thematic Dimension 6

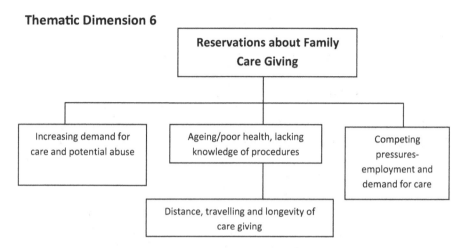

Increasing Demand for Care and Potential Abuse

The study found that some service users had a good relationship with their caregivers (e.g. SU5, 14, 15), but were afraid that increasing demand for care could exacerbate abuse of some sort, such as physical or emotional abuse, which could jeopardise family relationships. Some family caregivers could exaggerate care package with the intention to earn more money from social services. A large number thought that living together with the older relative was likely to intensify family dynamics and conflicts between siblings and the cared for person (e.g. SU6, 14, 15). The aftermath could be damaging to the philosophy of family care giving and families would fall apart and go their own ways, leaving social services to assume all responsibilities for continuing care. Some participants wished to see their families united and were supportive without a barrier. Families did quarrel and settled their differences but there was no perfect family system (SU15). The vignette commentary below helps to illustrate some of the views.

> Caring can be very demanding, this could increase both physical burden and stress, therefore resulting to frustration, and some form of abuse... I have been a carer I know what is like...and what Maggie is going through (SU6).

I mean some people are born carers and they feel, this is my responsibility, and I really must do this, but if she is resentful of it, that's not going to get any better, so a lot depends on the relationship between John and Maggie (SU8).

I think that is the key, what is the relationship between John (father and daughter) and Maggie, but I don't think money is the answer; there is potential...abuse there (SU15).

Ageing/Poor Health, Lacking Knowledge of Procedures

A large number (8/15) of the service users identified ageing and poor health as issues of concern for family care giving. Some recognised the impact this would have on them during care giving. A high proportion of the carers may lack the knowledge of assessment and legislative procedure to guide them as a result they would find it depressing to continue care giving. Most family caregivers were spouses, daughters, sons and daughters-in-law, while some of them were older people themselves with poor health (e.g. SU1, 3, 5). A number of them thought that these factors could potentially present some difficulties to continuing care, yet, irrespective of their age or poor health, they preferred to receive care from their relatives, supported by social services as appropriate.

My wife is 83 and she is my main carer, she has her own health problem, I wonder how she keeps on going... She does every thing for me but I am worried how long she could cope with this. I cannot rely on her...if she becomes ill, what can I do...? (SU6).

Competing Pressures Employment and Demand for care

Most participants (13/15) argued that care giving for an older relative was a big undertaking. Some (e.g. SU1, 2, 14) revealed that the younger members of the family would not be able to take on such responsibility for a longer time because they were either in full-time or part-time employment or running their own business. Although they received care from their relatives, they sometimes felt isolated and lonely when their relative went to work. Sometimes no family members were around to talk and socialise with them and this tended to upset them and could make them feel anxious and overwhelmed by an uncertain future (e.g. SU 6). They sometimes attempted to undertake some of their own care needs with extreme difficulty and this made them consider receiving care from social services instead of the family. Constant demand for care could have some ramifications on the family caregivers:

I live with my daughter with her children and they all work full-time. They are always tired when they come back from work and they had to provide care for me, it can be difficult for all of us and you could see the stress on their faces (SU3)

The pressure of keeping full-time job and caring for me can be profound on my family, even as I live with them, you could see tension bulling in the air, I think it's difficult sometimes... (SU5).

You're most of the time alone in the house when they go to work and you try to do some thing for yourself...that can be very difficult for me (SU6).

Distance, Travelling and Longevity of Care Giving

There was an acknowledgement by the majority of this group (11/15), which stated that long term care giving would not only increase demand for care but it could also induce stress or frustration because it seemed there was no end in sight (SU5, 6, 14 and 15). The caregivers may be travelling distances to provide care or to offer support to the best of their abilities and they are often tired. When this happened, it would affect their cordial relationship and care might break down. Some argued that many families would like to avert this situation from arising (e.g. SU2, 9, 10). Most argued that care giving could be a period of uncertainty and irritability and that little misunderstanding could aggravate arguments and conflict. A number alluded that people are living longer, their demand for care could be high, and not many family caregivers would cope for as long as it takes. The vignette responses illustrate the issues surrounding long term care giving:

Well, Maggie is going to be a prisoner nearly, in her own home, if she's got him in her own home, she's going to be a prisoner, as John might constantly be at her beck and call... that's the only difficulty I can see... with long term continuing care (SU5).

Obviously because she's got the responsibility, ultimately she's got the responsibility hasn't she, so from her point of view, there must be, because it must curtail her social life, and a lot depends of course on her age. She's 58, well that's the time when really you should have freedom, whether she's been married and had a family or not, I don't know she can cope looking after her father this is a difficult one... isn't it? (SU10).

My daughter travels long distance (five miles) daily to assist me. She is always tired and we some times quarrelled for little or no reason, I know how difficult it might be for her...you know I am 83 and how long would she continue to care for me? (SU11).

Conclusion

On reflection over two third of the participants (11/15) indicated that they would prefer their family members to provide care for them and they gave reasons such as knowing the care provider, shared values and family norms, respecting dignity and maintaining quality and standards of care. On the other hand, the study identified diverse and mixed views from the service users regarding their care needs. These findings are an insight into the feelings and expectations of older people towards who would assist them and attend to those needs. Focusing on the themes such as emotional, practical tasks, enabling support systems and socio-economic dimensions, a large number (7/15) of the group express some reservations about family care giving and felt that the proposed care model may have some consequences on the family. However, most thought that family care assessors/caregivers should be paid for their time and efforts committed during care giving. A significant minority of the participants (4/15) expressed concerns about reciprocal family care giving for payment. They stated that the model is a recipe for interference with their family members and therefore they would not like their family members to be involved in their care. Some of the service users expressed some reservations about the proposed care model of family care giving and thought that family structure is changing to smaller units. The changing family units have a significant influence on family-directed support care systems in the long run.

Chapter Four (B):
The Family Caregivers' Views

Introduction

The views of the family caregivers are crucially important to the outcome of this study. Their views demonstrate in part the rationale behind family care needs assessment and care giving as well as the advantages and disadvantages of the family-directed support care system. The study identified five key thematic dimensions with wide-ranging categories that are interrelated and distinctive to family care giving. Like with the service users' views, the analysis is based on core themes, which centred on family care giving, home care and older people who are the recipients of care from their family. The study also revealed three factors that are likely to influence family care giving: payment to family care assessors/caregivers, emotional and practical tasks, as well as enabling support systems.

The core and influencing factors are repeated in this chapter to draw a comparison between the views of the service users and the family caregivers such as daughters-in-law, spouses, daughters and sons. The similarities and differences will help in discussing the advantages and disadvantages of family care giving later in the thesis. The analysis provides inside knowledge of the family caregivers' world, their experiences and the rationale for their willingness to offer continuing care to older relatives. The analysis is illustrated by the extracts from the data in which the interviewees expressed their experiences and knowledge of care giving.

Their comments and quotations centred on inter-subjective perspectives, which help to clarify situations that could deflect or support their enthusiasm for care giving. The analytical process gives an account of the author's journey throughout the study, working with the family caregivers, listening to their experiences. This knowledge helped him to balancing his theoretical and practice-based understanding of social policy for older people. He was in a position to relate, gather accurate information from the participants and interpret it for clarity and simplification of the analysis, the family caregivers are coded as FG.

The study has shown that family care giving is central to preserving the family care continuum and reciprocity. It also involves the family participating in the assessment of care needs and care giving for their older relatives. These undertakings would enhance interaction between the family caregivers and their older relatives during care giving. Care giving carries with it emotional and practical care elements that have the potential to influence commitment as well as the ability to enhance continuing care. Emotional and practical dimensions work in parallel and complement each other, and the boundaries between them are sometimes difficult to establish during care giving. In this context, family-directed support care giving is divided into two thematic dimensions: emotional and practical. The thematic framework below identifies a number of categories that support the themes.

Emotional Dimensions

Emotional care is about making sure that older relatives feel that their psychosocial care needs are met with respect and dignity, and they are valued as people and treated as individuals whose care is being provided holistically by those who share the same values and belief systems. Care giving would mean something different at different levels of the family unit. The study identified that most of the caregivers are spouses or daughters. Each of them viewed their roles and expectations differently. The study revealed that care giving encompasses emotional and psychological qualities that could affect outcome. The study found that most of the group members (11/13) wished to provide care and a quarter illuminated different opinions. The Thematic Dimension Seven illustrated the themes and categories for this group:

Thematic Dimension 7

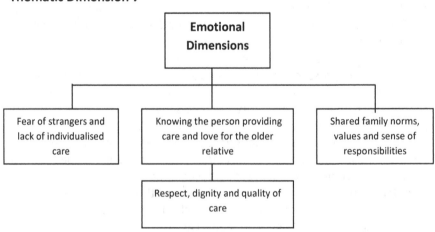

Fear of Strangers and lack of Individualised Care

Most family caregivers thought that some strangers could not be relied upon and expressed some concerns stating lack of experience, different carers at different times as a result they were unable to provided individualised care for the older relative. The majority (11/13) believed that some strangers cannot be trusted and may not have the experience to provide person centred care to older relatives who may be frail, disabled, and incapacitated to fend off abuse from strangers. A number (e.g. FG4, 7, 8, and 13) felt that trusting the lives of their older relatives in the hands of strangers is worrying as a result they would prefer to assist older relatives with their care. Some contended that older relatives deserved personalised care rather than seeing them as homogeneous care recipients without distinction.

> Oh it's obviously concerning and worrying... I mean we trundle along together, we don't do much because he doesn't want to do anything, he'd rather sleep all day if he had his choice... I made sure his care is provided the way he would have done it himself. You cannot trust strangers because you don't know them and some of them cannot be relied upon (FG1)

> I feel happy looking after them, because they're my parents... and I look after them, as well as my sisters. I don't like to see them struggle. I support them emotionally really. I see them every week, usually speak to them on the phone once or twice a week and strangers cannot assume this responsibility (FG3).

Knowing the Person Providing Care and Love for the Older Relative

Almost all the group members (11/13) stated that they had always looked after their older relatives without much help from social services and they would like to see this practice continue uninterrupted. Knowing the person providing care promotes care acceptance and reduces anxiety on the cared for person. There was a link between love and guilt and they could not abandon their older relatives when they needed them most. Participating in care giving helped some family members to understand themselves better and be able to provide holistic, as well as reciprocating to older relatives during care giving. This attitude helped to keep some families together and knowing the person providing care reduces the possibility of care breakdown (FG6, 7, 11). The study revealed that the period of care giving was often a time when some families came together and shared their grief, happiness and solidarity with one another. This could provide an opportunity to talk about family issues and to agree on how best to assist their older relatives. (FG1, 2, 6, and 10):

> Yes... like my grandmother, I used to go to her every day... it's just what we expect. Mum's care has brought us together once again and has made us stronger than ever before... I know many people... my sister-in-law does a lot of care for her mum and dad, friends of mine do a lot of care for their parents, so it's still there and that's the Irish way... (FG7).

Shared Family Norms, Values and Sense of Responsibility

The study also revealed the link between care giving, sense of responsibility and feelings of guilt if older relatives were not helped with their care needs. Most participants (11/13) thought that responsibility and a feeling of guilt to be inseparable and they overwhelmingly professed that they had a duty to provide care as and when needed. A number of them stated that they couldn't walk away from care giving (e.g. FG1, 2, 4). Shared family norms and values is one way of reciprocating to older relatives' support system. Most revealed that they had a good rapport and relationship with their older relatives, had shared their lives with them, and that the only way to show their appreciation was by taking part in their care. Some thought that their older relatives would be able to cope better emotionally with their difficulties during care giving. It was also about recognising the part that older relatives had played in their upbringing and the support they had given to their nuclear or reconstituted family when they had been fit and able to do so (e.g. FG1, 3, 8, 11).

> Any time they need me, I make every effort to see them irrespective of distance. I see their needs as mine, is a sort of paying back what they did for me and I will do every thing to support them for as long as possible. I see it as a duty and responsibility that I have to accomplish (FG2).

> My parents did give my brother and I all their love and they still give their whole support despite frailty and age. They will feel disappointed if we are unable to support them now they need us most. I don't think that I can live with such guilt and that will haunt me, it is a responsibility... (FG8).

Respect, Dignity and Quality of Care

A high proportion (11/13) of the family caregivers said that care giving was a process of taking over someone's life because of disabilities and deterioration in their health or wellbeing. For them this was about safeguarding dignity, respect, and providing quality care they deserved. Most (e.g. FG5, 9, 12, and 13) asserted that being part of the care giving process guaranteed that their older relatives would be treated with respect and quality of care assured. The majority stated that they had to respect their older relative's wishes. Although this could be difficult sometimes, they had to abide by their rules. Most thought that respect was not a skill that could be learnt easily but an instinct inherited from childhood, which formed part of their humanitarian skills. By respecting their dignity, they would feel valued and that would enable them to relax and be able to participate in the care process. Participation would help reduce frustration as well as aggression toward caregivers during care. Respect for dignity was seen as fundamental to each individual, some stated that their primary mission was to ensure their older relatives were happy, and respected during care giving.

My mum is a very shy woman who likes to preserve her privacy and dignity. She will be very reluctant to receive care... you know personal care from strangers... She feels happy for me to assist her knowing that I am her daughter and we share everything in common as a family. She does not resent me, I respect her wish, and I make sure that her dignity is respected at all time... (FG5).

Well, one important thing is there is consistency... it helps him keep his privacy and independence, his dignity, plus as father and daughter... it allows him to remain in his own home. If he's been unwell I have stayed the night, and I am going to hospital with him for three days and stay. I respect him for who he is despite frailty and ageing (FG9).

My father is a man who likes to keep things in a particular way in the house. He expects people to respect his wishes and observe his rules and principles. He feels that strangers would not adhere to his ways of life. He expects us to care for him knowing that we are aware of his expectations and will respect... you know... (FG10).

Practical Tasks during Care Giving
The study revealed that both the service users and carers had similar views about the practical aspects of care giving, which encompassed the interaction between the cared for person and caregiver during care and

which helped to promote psychosocial wellbeing between them. It is about the engagement of the family caregivers to assist their older relatives complete those physical functional activities, which they would be unable to accomplish because of ageing or ill health. The majority of this group (9/13) expressed their commitment to assist their older relatives with practical tasks. For some it was about continuous assessment, maintaining duty and responsibility, consistence of care giving, interdependence. However, one quarter (4/13) expressed different views see below. Thematic Dimension Eight illustrates the categories in more detail:

Thematic Dimension 8

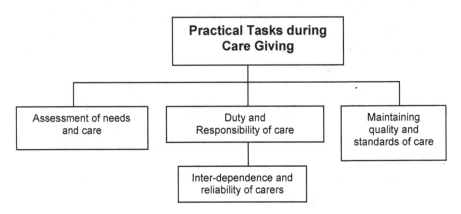

Assessment of Needs and Care

A large number of the group (9/13) indicated a wish to undertake care needs assessment. It was felt that such an assessment was a medium that enhanced personalised care packages, which would meet both emotional and practical care giving tasks. One of the cornerstones of family care giving was being responsible and partaking in assessment and care. For most family caregivers' needs assessment and care giving were about taking an active part, being responsible and carrying out daily care duties as necessary, whilst liaising with their older relative and other contributors to care giving (e.g. FG4, 7 and 13). The family caregivers knew and understood the needs of their older relatives better than any one else and were in a better position than social care workers to carry out care needs assessment. Their inside knowledge gave them the opportunity to identify and provide tailor-made support services. Over one half believed that social workers could not realistically capture the holistic needs of their older relatives within one or two hours of needs assessment. Assessment was a process and not a snapshot task as it took longer time to identify actual and potential needs. A large number of the family caregivers contended that assessment was an ongoing process. Some said family caregivers were better placed to carry out a realistic assessment of needs.

I think I am in a position to assess her needs and draw up a flexible programme of care that would meet her needs. I don't think that social workers would understand my mum's needs by just spending one or two hours assessing her needs... that's not realistic (FG7).

By contrast, a significant few (4/13) felt that assessment should be a joint approach between social workers and the family and/or older relative. They thought that this approach would provide broader decision making in identifying needs and drawing up a care plan that would reflect a holistic approach to activities of daily living. Social workers are independent of the family and their professional opinion and knowledge would be necessary to see beyond the family's personal views.

I think a joint assessment between social workers and the family would yield a better care plan. Families can only see... and their emotion and guilt could blight their decision making process during assessment and care. Social workers are trained professionals and could see things differently (FG10).

Duty and Responsibility of Care

The study revealed how deeply families are committed to care giving, despite pressures from different directions (e.g. nuclear family, employment). The study established that care giving was seen to be a responsibility and responsibility was synonymous to duty of care (FG4, 9, 13). Being responsible for their older relatives care needs made some family caregivers feel to be part of the decision making about arranging and providing care. The support they gave helped to ensure that older relatives were not lacking or being deprived of any essential assistance necessary to enhance wellbeing. Some indicated that they shared the duties and responsibilities amongst the entire family and sometimes spoke with one voice to social services and other supporting agencies as and when appropriate. The majority (8/13) felt obliged to fulfil these duties and responsibilities and they derived satisfaction in discharging them:

Mostly it's looking after things in the flat; you know cleaning surface and floor, and cleaning out her budgerigar, because she is not able to do that sort of thing any more... I do her hair... she manages to wash and dress herself at the moment, although when she is not feeling well I assist with personal care. I see these as my responsibility moreover as the only child... (FG4).

You know... I feel it is a duty and being responsible to look after her 24 hours a day, that's what I would prefer to do... generally... she can still wash her upper half... just making sure her feet and legs are cleaned daily because she's got diabetes and her skin is quite thin, just doing everything that she needed doing at that time (FG7).

In contrast, a significant minority (5/13) differed in their opinion from the majority's views and thought that duty and responsibility is in the eyes of the beholders. Families are different and would see things differently depending on their family cohesion. Family care giving cannot be imposed to the younger family members; they have their own family to care for as well as providing for themselves, otherwise the demand to care for older relatives could be overwhelming to bear.

I do their shopping for them, their housework and recently the gardening. I assist them with a bath once a week when I visit to see them. I don't see these as my duty and responsibility to support them for as long as possible. I do this in order not to be blamed by my other relatives; I have my own life to live... (FG10).

Maintaining quality and Standards of Care
The study showed that care giving required a degree of commitment to maintain quality standards throughout care giving period. Breakdown in care could affect the older relative and the entire care system. Almost all the group members echoed this (10/13). Some (e.g. FG1, 6, 10, 11) made references to their disappointment and experiences of poor quality of care that social service's care workers provided for their older relatives. Being part of the care system helped to ensure consistency and quality standards as to reduce the incidence of care breakdown (FG3, 7, 8). This gave the older relatives the confidence that their care needs would be provided for as and when necessary. It was argued that caregivers had the opportunity to plan ahead and make contingency plans to cover holidays, evenings and nights out without a breakdown in the care system.

Any breakdown in care will be devastating for him and I do my best to ensure that his needs are met at all times. My father is from the old school type and wants everything to be provided with out obstacle and I can't afford to let him down, he knows I am there for him (FG6). . However, a few (3/13) thought that quality standards are only subjective as people perceives quality differently. What is important during care giving is the assurance that essential care needs are met as appropriate and they are not exposed to danger or risk of harm in their own home:

> My parents used to have social services carers, but they never turned up most of the time and also they never phoned to say they are not coming... you know my parents had to phone me for assistance (FG9).

> We do our best to support my father, the most important thing is that he gets washed, housework can wait for another day and my father doesn't care about that ... (FG11).

> My parents are not overly bothered about the quality of their care...we try to help as we can... the main thing is that they are not in danger or at risk (FG2).

Inter-dependence and Reliability of Carers

The study uncovered the relationship between care giving and interdependence between the older relatives and their family caregivers. A number of caregivers (e.g. FG5, 6, 8, and 12) said that being part of their older relatives care made it easier to depend on one another and share their difficulties as well as supporting themselves. Informal care giving arrangement is more reliable than direct provision that was arranged by social services. They acknowledged that people were individuals with limitations. As a result, they depended on one another to guide themselves through difficult times. Most (10/13) argued that sharing accommodation with the older relative increased the propensity to rely on one another without asking outside help to achieve their holistic needs. Some expressed the difficulties an informal support system could impose on the stronger member of the cohabitation despite associated advantages (FG2, 7, 13).

> We've lived together for quite a long time and throughout this period we have always done things together helping one another and we manage our affairs. Now he can't do much but we still manage together. I cook our meals and I assist him some times with his wash, the only problem is my own health... you see I am diabetic... (FG6).

In contrast, a minority of the family caregivers (3/13) highlighted their difficulties and thought that placing older relatives in a residential or nursing home would be more accommodating to the entire family system. They expressed the view that social services should be fully responsible for older relatives' care needs and not the family, giving the complexity associated with long-tern care giving.

> Interdependence is only subjective and sometimes cannot be measured. For me it's an art and not science, people struggle together... and social service can help if it's within their criteria (FG11).

Enabling Support Systems

The growing older people population and their increasing demands for care have meant that all the participants (13/13) of the family caregivers were finding it increasingly difficult to cope without adequate back-up systems from social services. The study exposed some compelling enabling resource factors that could assist family caregivers to continue care giving for their older relatives for as long as possible. Some participants argued that undue pressures on them would potentially be reduced if these support systems were available and accessible. For some it would also help to maintain a safer environment and promote independence. Most caregivers would welcome assistance and support from social services or other family members to enable them continue care giving to older relatives in their own home. Thematic Dimension Nine below shows the advantages of enabling support services for the benefit of the cared for person and the family caregiver.

Thematic Dimension 9

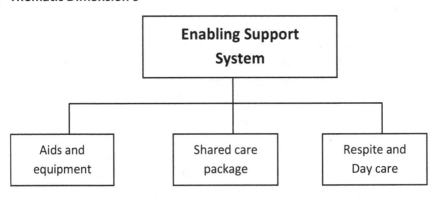

Aids and Equipment

The relationship between aids and equipment and long-term care were evident in the study. All group members (13/13) saw aids and equipment as a critical success factor for continuing care. Aids and equipment not only promoted the independence of the users but also helped family caregivers to undertake tasks such as manual handling, transfers, hoisting and lifting the older relatives without physically hurting themselves (FG3, 9, 12). It was thought that having access to aids and equipment such as commodes, walking frames, stair lift and grab rails would undoubtedly prolong care giving and independence. Availability of aids and equipment would give both the older relatives and caregivers the confidence to have

near independent living and less dependence on social services whilst risks are minimised. Most participants (e.g. FG1, 6, 9, and 11) argued that aids and equipment would reduce the incidence of falls and fractures, which were likely to occur during care giving:

> We could have relatively good quality of life if I could wheel him out of the house a couple of times a week to see some of our friends. We need a ramp to be able to get out, but social services do not see that need as essential (FG3).

> I think within social services, if you require, which we have done, a piece of equipment, the wait is far too long. And we've waited up to 14 weeks for a commode, which is totally unacceptable (FG9).

> My father is a big and tall man. Our social worker referred him for Occupational Therapy assessment for raised chair and bed. This equipment I hope would help me transfer him easily without much pressure on my knees and back, but we have waited for the equipment for a long time now... (FG10).

Shared Care Package

Although a high proportion of the caregivers (9/13) clearly stated their commitment to family care giving, some thought that having a split care package with social services would improve care giving (e.g. FG5, 8, 10). A split care package would give them the opportunity to concentrate on those tasks, which they had the skills and confidence to deliver without much difficulty. A shared care package would reduce pressures and the anxiety of rushing around trying to support older relatives. Shared packages of care would also give them the opportunity to devote some time to see to the needs of their nuclear or reconstituted families. This would give them more time to socialise with their family and plan together for the benefit of all family members (e.g. FG3, 11, 13). For them shared packages of care with social services would help to relief pressures upon them and could give them the opportunity to make long-term plans:

It was either myself or my husband was spending our time providing care to my mother-in-law, in the end the palliative nurses stepped in and it was wonderful to have them around... they did arrange... It was just having some space for yourself and your immediate family (FG8).

One thing I needed is a break during the day. Shared care package with social services would provide at least a sort of relaxation and to look after myself. Having him 24 hours, meeting all his care is very difficult and hard work to contain, as he is constantly demanding my time and presence (FG12).

In contrast, a significant minority (4/13) argued against shared care package with social services. They thought that share package would mean seeing different faces all the time and this would disorientate their older relatives more. Also they would like to preserve the respect and dignity for their older relative as they have standards and lifestyle they want to maintain till the end.

We have very good family relationships, my parents have had a high standard of living, and they would not like to see that interrupted. Split care packages with social services would not be acceptable to my parents, as they would not like to see different faces all the time... (FG7)

Respite and Day Care

Almost all the family caregivers (11/13) expressed their willingness to continue care giving to their older relatives, but stated that their lives would be more manageable if they had access to day and respite care as and when needed without restrictions. The findings echoed two important policy issues, namely social exclusion and resource limitation/rationing of services (e.g.FG1, 3). The study also uncovered that having access to resource centres would not only improve the quality and continuity of care, but would also help to reduce social exclusion and pressures on caregivers, as well as reducing the need for some older relatives to be placed or admitted into a residential care home (e.g. FG6, 10, 12). Respite or carers' breaks would help them regain and recuperate from their caring role and this would benefit all the stakeholders.

Without a support from social service, my life would gradually diminish within me; I think day care and continuous respite would mean a lot for me... (FG3).

Life would mean nothing without adequate carers' breaks... you know respite care and day care would be great and I can devote more time to care for her... (FG6).

Respite... that's the big thing, because my father goes to day centre twice a week... we are hoping that he goes for another day, but the big thing is respite so that my mother can get away completely or she's got a girlfriend that she sometimes goes on holiday with... I think that's the biggest thing (FG12).

Socio-economic Dimensions

The study highlighted that carers are individuals with developed personal lifestyles such as owning and running a car and paying a mortgage. This meant that some of them had to work longer hours and sometimes had two jobs to achieve their objectives. Meeting these demands in conjunction with care giving to older relatives could sometimes be more challenging than straightforward care giving. Combining care giving with other functional activities could result in conflicting demands on them and create a stressful and even physical burden. The majority (9/13) of the family caregivers found it increasingly difficult to combine these demanding tasks and they felt that payment of some sort would help to reduce the pressure on them.Almost one quarter (4/13) did not share this view and expressed their disagreement of paying family caregivers. Thematic Dimension Ten below exemplifies some of the views expressed by the family caregivers.

Thematic Dimension 10

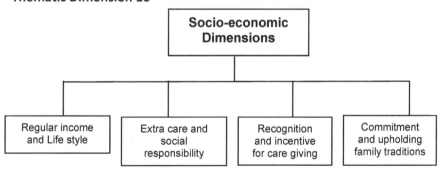

Regular Income and Lifestyle

The majority (9/13) of the group thought that payment would help some of the family caregivers to reconsider other personal engagements that contributed to lack of time and an inability to respond as and when required. Payment would provide a financial status that would assist them to sustain their own lifestyle such as mortgage and holidays. They would also be in a better position to tolerate the stress and pressure associated with care giving. Payment was not the decisive factor for some of the group members. The study found a multiplicity of factors linked with care giving: love, guilt, blame, choice and paying back the care and support older relatives gave to them from childhood. Changing economic circumstances meant that payment would help redress some of the family caregivers' socio-economic factors that could interrupt their commitment to care giving. By contrast, about one quarter (4/13) argued that payment to family caregivers might relegate family relationships. Reciprocal family care giving could not mix with financial rewards, as it would be immoral to do so:

> I will like to be paid for care that I am giving to my parents. You know I have a mortgage and my children are still dependent on me. I can't give all the time my parents require and at the same time, work to support my nuclear family. Payment towards the care that I give to my parents will be helpful I mean... (FG3).

> I think that I need regular income to sustain my livelihood and at the same time caring for my dad. We all need money to maintain our lifestyle don't we...? I care for my dad yet I still have to earn a living; it's difficult you know to juggle with the two... (FG9).

> I resent family members being paid for the care they give to their older relatives. I cared for my mum until she died and I never dreamt of being paid for it and I am now caring for my father, I will not like to be paid; it is a duty and paying back (FG12).

Extra Care and Social Responsibility
Extra income could be used to buy in extra care packages to support the family caregivers when they were unable to attend to their older relative's care needs (e.g. FG5, 9, 11). Over one half of the participants argued that extra income could be used flexibly for different tasks at different times during care giving. A large number (9/13) affirmed that payment would give them the opportunity to be creative and innovative and to offer holistic care to older relatives as and when necessary. It was also about lateral thinking and seeing care giving from a different perspective, and making alternative arrangements to meet future care

needs and demands. The findings showed that extra income would reduce constant demands on the family, as well as reducing the possibility of care breakdown, which could lead to residential care placement or intervention by social services. Although some family caregivers (4/13) recognised the importance of extra income, they were not of the view that this was the right approach to support their older relatives. Some thought that family reciprocity was about negotiating care responsibilities within the family and seeking assistance from social services as and when necessary:

> I think carers should be paid, and it shouldn't be taxable, and I also think there should not be any means testing. You can map yourself out a little bit more... I mean if you've got money for somebody to come in and bath him, and spend an hour doing this and that with him... (FG3).

> Extra income is rewarding, because it does help, I mean that does bring a lot of help to people... and of course, it does save a lot of worry because you do worry financially... you know (FG11).

> Family care giving is about sharing care responsibilities, seeks for help from social services as, and when appropriate. I don't believe that extra income is necessary for buying an extra care package. I reject any form of formal payment to family members (FG5).

Recognition and Incentive for Care Giving

Almost three quarters of the group (9/13) argued that payment for care giving to older relatives did not only offer the opportunity for extra income, but it was also about recognising the input families were making towards care giving for their older relatives (FG10, 11). Irrespective of the level of payment they received, some reaffirmed that they would continue to offer support. Payment would make them feel recognised by the social services that would otherwise pay strangers to provide care for their older relatives (e.g. FG7, 9, 12). Recognition was about appreciating the contributions the family caregivers made and would encourage them to commit more of their time and effort for the wellbeing of their older relatives.

> To pay carers yes, but what matters most is to recognise their contributions to uphold the wider welfare state, otherwise the state have to pay formal carers, who are in my opinion unprofessional in their approach Best Value concept (FG5).

In my opinion, payment is synonymous to recognition of the contributions that family members make towards the welfare service. Given their own economic wellbeing I feel that payment would be advantageous to some families to remain loyal and continue offering care to their older relatives (FG9).

However, a significant minority (4/13) argues against the care model. Most contended that family care giving was a duty the younger members of the family owed their older relatives. It would be ill thought of the family caregivers to expect their efforts to be financial compensated by the state. Social services were there only as an enabler and should only interfere when the family was not coping and should not to take over the family's responsibilities (FG4, 5, 7). Some said it was unethical and they could not compromise their conscience despite the difficulties and pressures upon them and their family. Payment would not be a substitute for the love they had for their older relatives.

I recognized the economic impact on some of the family carers, but I cannot envisage the reasons to be paid for caring for my mother. I admit it is difficult to provide care, but it is part of paying back... otherwise what is the family about. It will be meaningless... I cannot compromise with that.... No, I'll not support payment to family carers. Well family care has been part of my family belief and I cannot change that belief for cash... (FG6).

Commitment and Upholding Family Traditions
Almost all the family caregivers contended that continuing care for older relatives required a commitment of time and effort and this would not come cheap (e.g. FG10, 11). Family care giving has been part of their family reciprocated cycle and continues to revolve and evolve from one generation to another and they are committed to preserve this heritage. However, over one half (7/13) had their nuclear or reconstituted families to support. Most stated if they had known in advance that they would be paid for caring, they would have prepared themselves better knowing that at the end they would be paid. This understanding would have given them the opportunity to plan and prioritise their activities and be in a better position to carry out care in a more organised and efficient way. Many argued that combining care giving to older relatives and trying to meet the needs of their nuclear/reconstituted families could put unbearable pressure on them (e.g. FG2, 8, 13):

We live in a very materialistic society and we all need money to secure our livelihood, as a result it will be difficulty to commit yourself caring for your older relatives without payment. I mean commitment goes along with financial remuneration... (FG7).

To be honest, I think carers should be paid because if he were living in a residential care home, it would cost the government a lot of money. So yes, it will be easy to manage and you are in control of the care giving, unlike what we have now from the care agencies... that never turn up sometimes... and would not even be bothered to phone... What many carers want is a wage and they can commit themselves to care for their older relatives (FG12).

Reservations about Family Care Giving

The study uncovered wide-ranging issues and concerns that could influence some family caregivers' decisions about whether to continue care giving, despite their enthusiasm to assist their older relatives. Care giving could be very demanding on caregivers and their nuclear or reconstituted families. A large number of the group (7/13) said they were affected physically, emotionally, and economically. As a result, deciding whether to participate in care could be difficult for many of them. Despite their reservations, about a half (6/13) felt that it was a duty they had to fulfil until the end, irrespective of the difficulties. Thematic Dimension Eleven explores the difficulties facing many family caregivers.

Thematic Dimension 11

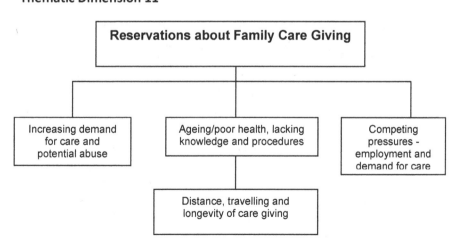

Increasing Demand for Care and Potential Abuse

A high proportion of this group (10/13) asserted that care giving could be very demanding and could change family relationships, behaviour and attitudes to a great extent, and that could affect one's approach to care and coping mechanisms. Some stated that constant demands on them could lead to abusive situations such as physical, deprivation and negligence and these could lead to a breakdown in support systems. Most (e.g. FG8, 11, 13) expressed their commitment to care giving and highlighted that their primary aim was to ensure their older relatives were looked after properly. Many family caregivers used terminology like "perseverance" and "exercising self-control" during care giving to justify their commitment and the high level of self-control they had to observe during care giving:

> I understand the difficulties surrounding care giving and am committed to it. It's my promise to my both parents that I will support them until the end... but it's a very difficult decision and choice... I enjoy the challenge, but it's very stressful and time consuming... you know but..., you could lose your temper, and that could be regarded as abuse or something else... (FG2).

> Look, don't forget we're all humans and we can easily lose our temper due to frustration and constant demand on your time, energy and person. Such pressures could lead to either physical or emotional abuse or total breakdown in care giving. I think is a question of perseverance and exercising personal control to avoid abuse of any kind... it could be very frustrating you know... (FG13).

Ageing/Poor Health and Lacking Knowledge and Procedures

Care giving involved emotional and physical wellbeing to meet the challenges that could be imposed on caregivers (FG3, 8, 9). It was argued by some that ageing and deterioration in their own health could be issues of concern to continuing care (FG7, 10). In as much as you would like to support, you may not have the necessary knowledge and skills to adopt the legislative guidance and procedures and as a result you are leaving yourselves open to criticism when things go wrong. Almost all (11/13) the group were spouses, daughters and daughters-in-law and some argued that although they were prepared to assist their relatives, they were also conscious of the impact it would have on their own health. Most said that for as long as their health would permit, irrespective of their age, they would continue to provide care (FG4, 7, 13).

My only problem is my own poor health... am not a well woman you know my health is dodgy... I have blood pressure and my hips aren't good as well so I can't do much for him, but am committed to continue... until I am unable to assist him, but it's not a simple task... (FG10).

We are committed to one another and he will do the same for... The only problem for me is that I am not young any more. I don't have the necessary skills and knowledge of legislation to guide me. I am nearly as old as he is (83); there is not much I can do; yet I will be there for him... (FG11).

Competing Pressures Employment and Demand for Care

Some group members expressed concerns about competing pressures on them. Some explained that they were finding it increasingly difficult to combine full- or part-time employment or business with care giving for their older relative and their nuclear family (e.g.FG5, 12). Some explained that these were two opposing factors, which sometimes stretched them beyond their capabilities. This affected their physical and psychological well-being as well as their relationship with their nuclear family (e.g. FG3, 8). They needed to be fit to be able to provide quality care. Some said they liked going to work and could not afford not to. Working in itself was stimulating and that helped them to cope with stress, as well as maintaining social contacts with colleagues and friends (e.g. FG7, 10). These perspectives brought to light issues such as social network outside care giving and lifestyle, which could be a measure to reduce stress levels:

I've got a full-time job and would not be able to travel to see them on a daily basis. That's the most important reason; I just couldn't afford full-time care giving to them... I work full time. I like going out to work; I like the challenge of my job, still I have to do my possible best to care for them... its hard (FG3).

I try to balance my life by making sure that I'm giving my grandchildren some attention... I never stop, I'm constantly on the go, even at weekends, but I think the major thing nowadays is, because people are living longer, you don't exactly catch up... of course you don't (FG7).

I think caring for your parents is a choice only you can make and hence you have made that choice and decision you have to carry it through... I work full time and combining care and employment is a very hard thing to do, but is a choice (FG10).

Distance, Travelling and Longevity of Care Giving

The study revealed difficulties that some family caregivers were having due to travelling long distances from one geographical area to another in order to provide care. Travelling every day before and after work for those who were still working affected not only their health but also their physical ability to provide care (e.g. FG6, 7, 13). Travelling made them tired and stressed and these situations could lead to unexplained arguments and conflict between the older relatives, other family members and themselves. Some asserted that even with improvements in transport systems, many of the caregivers were older themselves and felt that travelling, coupled with the physical nature of care giving, was not helping their enthusiasm for care giving. A number indicated that they have been caring for their older relative more than expected, but unsure how long care giving would continue (FG3, 8):

> To be honest I don't mind caring for mother but the problem is the distance that I have to travel on a regular basis. I don't drive, I travel by bus and some times buses are not regular, and you have to wait for a long time and that affects my ability and it increases my stress levels thinking how I am going to continue caring for her... (FG4).

> I am happy caring for my mum, she's in her 90s, and I am 74 this year. I travel 20 miles return every day to assist and be with her. You know travelling every day is tiring together with caring. I wish I could live with her but she refused to move in with me... I like caring for her but because of the distance and my own age I don't know how long... (FG5).

Conclusion

Family-directed support care system is seen by most carers as crucially important to safeguarding family norms and values and promoting family reciprocity in a post-modern era. This practice has restorative qualities that are not only beneficial to older people but equally to wider society. It gives the entire family the assurance that their older relatives are receiving adequate and quality care from people they are familiar with. The findings showed that over two thirds (9/13) of the family caregivers would like to undertake needs assessment and provide care. They cited various reasons such as feelings of guilt, feelings of love, respect and dignity, maintaining family norms and values, and maintaining family relationships. Although the majority was willing and committed, yet a large number (10/13) expressed their reservations about the difficulties of coping with continuing care for their older relatives. Nevertheless, the group was optimistic to continuing care for older relatives until they are unable to do so in future. The study identified a number of issues that are likely to influence decision making by many family caregivers either to abandon or limit their commitment to a family-directed support care system. The issues of concern are: 1) Ageing and poor health. 2) Competing pressures – employment and care giving to both nuclear/reconstituted family as well as older relative. 3) Distance and travelling to offer care to older relatives. At the same time, about a quarter (4/13) of the family caregivers stated that they would not accept a payment for caring for their older relatives. Some pointed out that they would feel guilty and believed that it was wrong and unethical to be paid for care giving for their older relatives.

Chapter Four (C):
Practitioners', Managers' and Councillors' views

Introduction

The study has focused on the viewpoint of key stakeholders about family-directed support care. It would be thus incomplete without the views of social services managers, social work practitioners and the county councillors who are at the forefront of formulating social care policies and commissioning social care packages for older relatives. This group's views are as important as other stakeholders – service users and family caregivers.

The data analysis is centred on three thematic dimensions: family care giving, assessment of older relatives' care needs, and payment to the family care assessors and caregivers. The approach is similar to that of the service users' and family caregivers' analytical dimensions, but differs in some aspects, mainly due to the fact that the group consists of three sub-groups: seven practitioners, four managers and two councillors, all with diverse views. They are grouped together because of their unique interest and representation within social services for example; policymaking, commissioning and assessment of care needs. The aim is to explore the views of each sub-group in-depth, in order to ascertain the differences and similarities of their opinions of the research questions.

This analytical process also examines the implications of the proposed care model for the county council and for the national government, as well as how to manage the scarce resources available for the growing older people population and their increasing need for care. It also considers the group's loyalty in terms of their political views, professional identity, and advocacy roles, protecting their job or career whilst serving the best interests of their employers.

The author used this chapter as part of his intellectual journey as a researcher rather than as a social worker-manager. In this context, he sought the views of his colleagues and employers whilst he carried the interviews in a professional manner without undue influence. He remained as consciously unbiased, factual and open to participants whilst asking probing questions in order to gather accurate and undistorted information to aid the development of a potential care model. This approach helped to generate themes upon which the analysis is based.

The following codes have been used: practitioners (P), managers (M) and councillors (CL). Family care giving is discussed by looking at the components of care giving, namely emotional needs and practical tasks during care giving. This thematic dimension presented in this chapter synchronises with those presented in the two previous chapters.

Emotional Dimensions

Meeting emotional need is one of the major issues that inspired family-directed support care systems. It is not only about making the older relatives feel valued and comfortable and removing fear of the unknown but also about believing and reassuring them that care giving would be provided unremittingly by people they know. As highlighted in the previous chapters, fear, anxiety and poor quality of care giving means that some older people may prefer to seek assistance from people they know rather than strangers. The thinking behind this concern is to maintain quality of care, participation and flexible care giving which it is hoped would improve the psychosocial wellbeing of all concerned.

The study showed that almost one half (3/7) of the practitioners, half (2/4) of the managers and one of the two councillors thought that family care giving would offer adequate emotional and psychosocial care. In contrast, over a half (4/7) of the practitioners, half (2/4) of the managers and one of the two councillors argued that social care workers were in a better position than family members to offer emotional care. A few practitioners stated that they were trained professionals and would therefore apply both theoretical and practice-based knowledge and experiences during care management. Thematic Dimension Twelve below identifies themes upon which the analyses are based:

Thematic Dimension 12

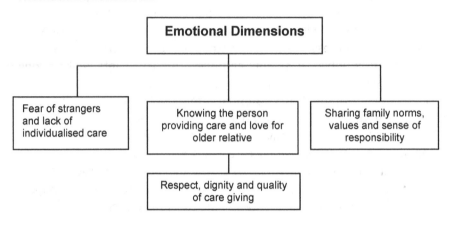

Fear of Strangers and Lack of Individualised Care
Practitioners' View

Following on from the previous views expressed, over one half (4/7) of the practitioners viewed individual care as important and argued that some family caregivers were able to offer more individualised care than strangers. The older relatives would be aware and understand that a holistic programme of care had been planned and provided by the family members (P7). This action plan reassured them that their care needs would be met, taking into account their specific needs. Older relatives would be seen as individuals and not as members of a group whose needs were met without due focus and attention to their specific requirements (P6). It was acknowledged that people were different in terms of individual needs and expectations. This perspective would counter the emphasis on homogeneity of care, which disregarded the unique requirements of the individual service user (P2).

> From my point of view, the advantages... are that the service user will be seen as an individual with certain needs and care will be tailored to meet those individualistic care needs. I don't think that strangers see beyond the boundaries of a care plan (P6).

Three practitioners did not share these views in full. Some (e.g. P3, 5) argued that social care for older people was implemented in line with legislation and policy guidance such as the National Service Framework for older people (DH 2001) and the NHS and Community Care Act (1990). Some of the practitioners highlighted the view that social services were committed to offer an individual care programme approach. However, social services had to provide care within resource availability (e.g. P1, 4). Given the growing older people population and increasing demand for care, the critical and substantial care matrix had to be applied; otherwise, social services would not be able to cope. Families had to take part in some form of social re-engineering in society and the wider welfare service.

> My view is that strict care needs assessment is the key critical success factor to uphold the welfare system in its present format and families have to be part of that social re-engineering... (P1).

Managers' View

Three out of the four managers thought that service user focus was a legislative requirement and therefore all service users should be seen as people with tailored care packages. They expressed the view that some families were well equipped to offer individualised care than strangers would. Some cited empathy, family links and guilt, as well as having a broader knowledge about their older relative and the world around them, as the reasons why the family members might offer a holistic package of care (e.g. M2, 4). Family caregivers could offer care beyond the care plan because of their closer relationship and fear of being blamed by other family members, or even the older relative. For them, emotional care was an integral part of holistic care giving. One manager thought that a user's focus sometimes went beyond what formal social care workers could offer, because of workload, budgetary constraints, and Fair Access to Care (M1). In contrast, one manager disagreed with the majority views and stated that social workers had to deliver care within resource availability. As a result, any assessment that was not within critical or substantial needs would be regarded as unmet need M3).

> Emotional care for older relatives is an integral part of holistic care giving. User focus sometimes goes beyond what the formal social care workers can offer because of workload, budgetary constraints, and Fair Access to Care (M1).

> As an informal carer, sometimes you take into account love, guilt as well as having broader knowledge about the cared for person and provide care to that person as an individual beyond what the strangers can... this is because you know them very well and what they wanted... (M4).

Councillors' View

Despite their differing political philosophies, both councillors saw user focus and individualised care as important for the wellbeing of the service users. Individualised care had the potential to reduce complaints, bad publicity against the council, wastage and duplication of care (CL1). The perspective would promote respect and dignity for the users and hopefully help them deal appropriately with their condition with less anxiety and fear of the unknown. Offering individualised care might also help the users to achieve their aspirations to be cared for in their own home for as long as possible (CL2). Both acknowledged, irrespective of political affiliations, that service user focus had political benefits and they referred to their loyalty to the electorate. They argued that a user focus was bipartisan and no political party would like to be the loser.

> In my opinion, you know... user focus has political benefits, irrespective of my political affiliation, which I strongly believe... we are accountable to the electorates... you can't mess them up... with their care... I mean you don't have to be righteous to realise that individualised care has the potential to reduce complaints, bad publicity against the council, wastage and duplication of care (CL1).

> The family should have a better understanding of their older relatives' needs... the small idiosyncrasies that that person has... and provision of care should be more focused because it is a family member and the person is not seen as a homogeneous product (CL2).

Knowing the Person Providing Care and Love for the Older Relative
Practitioners' View

The Majority of the practitioners (5/7) thought that knowing the person providing care and vice versa. Would promote continuity of care and this might help to establish a care pattern that met older people care in the long run. Some (e.g. P1, 3, 7) thought that family caregivers would not let their older relatives down. A comparison was drawn between family care giving and direct provision, which was characterised by poor time keeping, non-compliance to the care plan and lack of a designated key worker by some provider agencies (P4). In addition, some surmised that family care giving would sustain care giving in the long-term (P5, 7).

> You will always recognise your family and you will always rely on them for your needs, this cannot be the same with

strangers... Continuity to me is about having care continuum (P7).

A few practitioners (2/7) disagreed with the views expressed by the majority. They argued that quality of care depended on family relationships, culture and tradition (P6). They maintained that family circumstances (e.g. divorce, poor health) could prevent continuing care. Different circumstances would present different reactions and solutions to deal with or reduce the problems. What was important was the quality of care giving and that the service user was not at risk during care giving (P2).

Families are different at all levels, depending on family backgrounds, traditions and culture. Family problems such as divorce, childbirth and poor health of a caregiver could present different demands, and I think these could potentially affect continuity and consistency of care giving (P6).

Managers' View

Three of the four managers expressed the view that intimately knowing the caregiver was an important element of a holistic care package and this helped to calm the cared for person during care giving. Some argued that knowing the person providing care promoted rapport and co-operation between them. It also enhanced reliability, commitment and trust that were already established between them (M1). The older relatives were better off with their family caregivers than strangers because someone they knew very well would meet their needs and that person understood their needs (M4). Most family caregivers would always be available to support or share the responsibilities of care giving. This understanding would reduce anxiousness, communication breakdown and complaints between the caregiver and the cared for person/ families (M2, 4).

Knowing the caregiver would improve response time for care as well as assistance or support to cope with difficult situations during care giving. It would also reduce anxiousness, communication breakdown and complaints from the families (M2).

Councillors' View

The councillors were divided in their views. These were probably due to their political allegiances and socio-economic background. The councillor from the Right stated that knowing the person providing care would help to reduce anxiety and fear of the unknown. He pointed out that knowing the caregiver would enhance co-operation and long lasting relationships. For him this could also prevent conflict and breakdown in care giving. He also stated that knowing the caregiver could alleviate stress on the family as well as the cared for person.

> In an actual sense, I feel that knowing the caregiver would enhance participation during care giving. You know... knowing the person giving care would help to boost morale, confidence to cope and accept your condition better... For me it is about commitment and perseverance between the cared for person and the caregiver (CL1).

The councillor from the Left did not share this view but argued that the modern family was more complex compared to family care giving in the 1940s, 1950s and even 1970s. She stated that intimately knowing the person providing care couldn't be a qualification to re-dress fear of the unknown. She indicated that social services have a duty under legislation to meet the critical and substantial care needs of older people. She affirmed that knowing the caregiver was insignificant to continuity of care.

> The council is committed to quality of care giving besides who offers the care. We have both duty and power to provide care within budgets, and in accordance with the community care guidance, therefore it has to abide by that... and it is not interested about who the carers are... (CL2).

Sharing Family Norms, Values and Sense of Responsibility
Practitioners' View

The minority of the practitioners (3/7) thought that sharing family history was linked with the philosophy of knowing the caregiver providing care for an older relative. Family care giving would provide the forum for them to share ideas, their family history and belief systems (e.g. P2, 4). This understanding would help the older relatives to be composed and responsive to care giving. They did not have to explain themselves repeatedly to the caregiver as they probably would with strangers (e.g. P3, 5). Sharing family norms and history could be one of the ways to support themselves and cope well with the situations confronting them.

> Sharing family norms and values is about learning the family's past and adopting that belief system. I mean you cannot change people's belief from the way they do things (P2).

> Caring for your older relatives would provide a forum for the carer and the cared for person to see himself or herself as

one, talk about the family history, values and things that keep them together (P4).

However, a significant number (4/7) of practitioners argued that the family system was not static. Some said that families were changing in some respects. It was unrealistic to expect the traditional family system to remain unchanged in the present cultural diversity and approaches to life (P5). One stated; "The world is becoming a global village; culture and tradition is no longer fixed, but very fluid." (P7). One practitioner made references to the sociology and psychology of family theory and stated that after a period of time people (migrants) started to learn and adapt to a new culture and that they gradually abandoned their original culture and tradition (e.g. P3).

Behaviours and attitudes change overtime, depending on the dominant culture and traditions within the community and society. These I think affect or challenge traditional opinions, family norms and values. Politics and commerce have made the world a global village I think... (P3).

Managers' View

All four managers concluded that sharing family norms and history was one way to promote reciprocal family care giving in a way that was not threatening to the older relatives during care (M1). For them sharing family values would enhance an individualised care approach, would increase participation in care giving within the family, and, it was hoped, would help to develop a care pathway for the family and the generation that would come after them (M2). Sharing family history could also reveal some difficulties between now and in the past and, how they overcame their problems of care giving for their older relatives (M3). Sharing family values and belief systems for most would help to build family resilience against reliance on the state for health and social care needs (M4).

My belief is that most families have their preferences and approaches to care for the older relatives without relying on the state, and this is passed on between to generations (M2).

It's obvious that sharing family history could be the greatest teacher... You can only learn by examples and we have seen this amongst many communities and some religious groups in today's Britain... (M4).

Councillors' View

The findings also revealed the councillors' contrasting views about sharing family norms and values. One thought that sharing family values would promote emotional wellbeing during care. It was also a chain that linked quality of care, consistency and continuity of care as well as knowing the caregiver. He believed that family care giving would help to promote choice, control and wellbeing of the cared for person. For him family care giving would be a challenge to social services' unrealistic rationing of time for a care package and he cited examples of the 15 and 30 minutes care commissioning policy that was now prevalent among councils nationally.

> Current changes in social services are long overdue in my opinion... family care giving... is a new idea within the industry as I see it... It could bring about things like choice, control and a focus within the wider community care. Family care giving I hope would change the way we do things now and projects future social work and social care for service users... (CL1).

The perspective of the councillor from the Left contrasted with these views. She highlighted that the contemporary family system was diverse in attitude, behaviour and approaches to family support systems. She argued that the small family unit of today had reformed family support systems within an extended family. People were more individualised and offered assistance amongst themselves. The family was small in size and free to move around the globe to enhance social mobility, economic prosperity and even in search of employment and it was likely to adapt to that emerging culture and tradition. She affirmed that this changing attitude and a shrinking family unit placed social services in a unique position to be more responsible in line with legislation, to meet the growing older people population's care needs.

> Apart from politics, we all know that the family unit of today has eroded the historic extended family of the post-industrial... I mean, they are more individualised and concentrate their support system amongst themselves. They are free to migrate to other geographical areas in search of new life... (CL2).

Respect, Dignity and Quality of Care Giving
Practitioners' View

The study found that three out of the seven practitioners (3/7) expressed the view that family caregivers would offer quality care to their older relatives whilst their dignity is respected. The practitioners acknowledged that family care giving could lead to a higher quality of care compared to what strangers would offer under direct provision (e.g. P5, 3). They surmised that strangers might not have the extra time and capabilities to provide emotional care needs that were not tabulated in the care plan (e.g.P3, 4). For some practitioners, family caregivers had in-depth knowledge of their older relatives' aspirations and psychological needs and this would assure respect for dignity at all times.

> I feel that strangers are constrained by some factors such as time and probably inexperience, as a result they have different ideas of what is required to promote wellbeing and quality of care (P3).

> Strangers are paid workers; they don't have much time with regard to emotional care. They only focus on the care plan... Time constraint could inhibit the opportunity to respect user's dignity (P4)

However, over one half of the practitioners (4/7) expressed the view that maintaining respect, dignity and quality of care meant different things to different people and it could not be guaranteed even within the family. Some thought that family caregivers could equally offer poor quality of care (P1, 6). They that argued that respect for dignity and quality of care giving was associated with skills, knowledge and experience and felt that social care workers possessed these qualities more than some family caregivers. A number of them pointed out that most social caseworkers were highly qualified, trained and would offer holistic functional care to service users within the legislative framework (e.g. P2, 6).

> Social workers are trained and have wide-ranging experiences, knowledge and skills that cannot be compared with the family caregivers (P2).

> Maintaining respect, dignity and quality care giving cannot be guaranteed... it depends on skills, knowledge and experience of the caregivers. It would be over generalisation to think that all family members would observe respect, dignity and quality of care to older relatives (P6).

Managers' View

Two out of the four managers thought that family members had a holistic overview of the quality of life the service users were used to and were capable of respecting that during care giving (M3). One of the managers stated that strangers had a different idea of what was required to promote wellbeing, respect and dignity (M4). It was about promoting the psychological wellbeing of the cared for person. Strangers sometimes were only interested in meeting the needs outlined in the care plan and not concerned with psychological wellbeing of their clients. This is where their role as formal caregivers could not be equated to that of the family caregivers. Offering quality of care was an essential component of emotional care (M3).

> A family member is with that person and sees it from a much more personal level... you know sometimes family members have more of an overview of the quality of life the person has been maintaining. Strangers however may have a different idea of what is required... what his/her life should be or can be... so that would be good (M3).

The managers were divided in their opinion. The other two argued that social care workers were in a better position to offer quality care to their clients rather than family members. They highlighted that social care workers were independent of the cared for person and their family, therefore were in a position to offer care within Fair Access to Care and within the county council's social care policies (M2). Respecting dignity is subjective and immeasurable and that is the unmet need, which family members should attend to. It was stated that social services complied with the legislative care standards and frameworks and offered quality care as assessed by social workers, and monitored by the quality and development unit of the county council (M1).

> Good assessment and care encompasses a blend of policies, legislation and social work theory, and social workers are equipped with these knowledge-based values, therefore are well positioned to offer quality care to older people than their family members (M1).

Councillors' View

The councillors demonstrated their views in line with their political philosophies. The councillor from the Right was in favour of reciprocal family care giving and that embraces respecting the dignity of their older relatives. He expressed the view that the state could not continue to meet the entire health and social care needs of the growing older people population in the foreseeable future. He asserted that the family was better positioned to offer quality and psychological care to older relatives than the strangers. He referred to biological and cultural links between the families, their shared knowledge of care and history, which strangers lacked.

> In my opinion the family will not go wrong to an extent to offer emotional care to older relatives than strangers. They understand themselves better linked by biological and cultural links between them... their shared history is an advantage over what strangers could offer (CL1).

Conversely, the other councillor (CL2) argued that family care giving could not be relied upon. Some family members might have their own agenda and as a result might not have the time or opportunity to offer quality and psychological care. She argued that the state had set rules and approaches within its quality assurance frameworks to attend to the needs of the service users. She contended that "time and commitment" were an absolute necessity for quality of care and that the families of this era were busy and mobile and therefore did not have the time. She concluded that social care workers had all the qualities and professionalism to promote respect and dignity of the user whilst carrying out their tasks.

> The local authorities have policies and protocols that offer guidelines on assessment and criteria for care provision for service users. Social services would not solely depend on the family because some of them are busy and cannot commit themselves to care giving for a long time... we have a duty... you know (CL2).

Assessment Themes

It emerged from the study that family care giving might lead to a changing professional approach to social work in terms of assessment of needs, professional ethics and standards, family relationships and response to referrals for social care. In view of the issues raised, the three sub-groups had diverse opinions regarding the reciprocal family care giving approach and its contributions towards the existing service frameworks and the wider welfare system. Such concerns could present some obstacles and dilemmas for older people now and in the future. The findings showed that the majority of the sub-groups (5/7 practitioners, 3/4 managers, 1/2 councillors) were ambivalent about family members assessing the care needs of their older relatives. Thematic Dimension Thirteen below helps to unravel the views expressed by the sub-groups:

Thematic Dimension 13

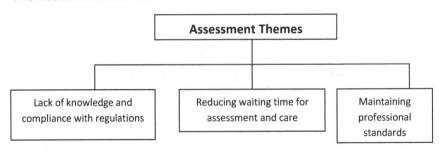

Lack of Knowledge and Compliance with Regulations
Practitioners' View

The quality of needs assessment was raised as an issue of concern by the majority (5/7) of this sub-group and a number of them stated that some family assessors would be unable to adhere to the National Care Standards when undertaking holistic assessment of needs (e.g. P4, 5). It would be difficult to monitor family care assessors in line with the policy and procedures outlined in the legislation. Implementation of the model could be flawed, thereby limiting compliance with the policy, as many of the family caregivers might not be able to interpret and abide by the policy and procedures (e.g. P1, 3, 6). A comparison was drawn between the proposed care model and the conventional care models. It was acknowledged that under existing care models of direct provision and direct payments, the quality and development team within the Essex County Council would carry out random annual checks of the quality of assessment by social workers (P1). Most argued that this process might not be permissible under the proposed care of family-directed support systems (e.g. P 4). Monitoring care giving for older relatives helped to uncover inconsistent care giving, as well as identifying those agencies that were not upholding the care regulations:

> My concerns are about compliance with legislation, policy and procedures as some family may lack the knowledge of legislation. I am not sure if many of the family members would understand or have the knowledge of these... probably not... I don't know (P3).

> As a provider one of my first issues is the National Care Standards... how the providers of care, albeit they are relatives, would still be assessing and providing care to an individual, to comply with the standards in a registered or regulated way... am not sure about that...(P5).

Managers' View

Three of the four managers (3/4) echoed the views expressed by the practitioners. Some said that social services had a duty under the legislation; the NHS and Community care Act (1990), to offer assessment within resource availability (e.g. M1, 3). Some pointed out that social services had a far greater requirement from a statutory point of view to be rigorous in assessment, bearing in mind the Fair Access to care eligibility criteria policy. Some commented that people who were trained should undertake assessment of care needs or experienced in care management, and not the family members, otherwise this could lead to a dereliction of duty. Some family caregivers may lack comprehensive knowledge of legislation and care standards approach (M2).

> I think we have got to actually draw the difference between what the families' capacity and implications are to what the county council as an authority are... Social services have a duty under the legislation and by allowing families to assess, to me... I mean it would mean abdicating responsibilities bestowed to it by Parliament; social workers have to focus their minds on Fair Access to care criteria (M2).

Councillors' View

Although one of the councillors acknowledged the difficulties associated with non-compliance with legislation during assessment by some family members, he nevertheless felt that many family care assessors might have good knowledge of legislation and the assessment process. He was of the view that, family care assessors had the potential to offer quality assessment to their older relatives. He thought that it was an exaggeration by the practitioners and some politicians to conclude that the family care assessors would not be able to comply with the National Care Standards. He stated that family care giving was an emerging strategic vision in the 21st century, which hopefully would ensure that the needs of the growing older people population were catered for in the community.

> My view is that there are some family members with potential to offer quality assessment to their older relatives of the type of care they wish to have, in their own home and in the community they are used to... We don't have to make blanket statements, condemning all family caregivers... (CL1).

By contrast, the other councillor argued that assessment and care giving could be a long-term commitment, depending on the nature of needs such as disabilities and degenerating ill health. Hence, it would be unethical to delegate responsibilities for assessment to the family members. Such conditions could aggravate situations that both the older relatives and the family assessors might find intolerable, depressing and challenging to cope with during care giving.

> Longevity of care giving could pose unbearable psychosocial conditions to both the cared for person and the family carers. Therefore undertaking needs assessment and care giving for their older relatives could increase the burden and stress of continuing care. However, assessment by social workers is impartial, independent and less traumatic to the service user and the family members (CL2).

Reducing Waiting Time for Assessment and Care

Practitioners' Views
Linking with the previous theme, a majority of practitioners (4/7) thought that family care giving would help bridge the gap between assessments and care provision (P4). A proportion of them echoed the views expressed by some of the service users and their caregivers. Many of the practitioners confirmed that waiting times for care packages could exacerbate anxiety and stress as well as psychosocial health problems for older relatives and their families (e.g. P2, 6). The majority thought that families undertaking needs assessment would provide an opportunity to rethink the roles and responsibilities of social care workers (P7).

> I think in terms of assessment, if we could get it right, it should help to bridge the gap. In theory if one of our relatives needed a service we would happily search around including the Internet, we would happily look for information, happily usually many of us fill in a form to get the ball rolling, and that would presumably help us as well and I think this reduces pressure on social workers (P7).

The minority (3/7) of the practitioners thought that family care giving was not the way forward to address waiting times for assessment and care packages. They argued that what was needed was a joint approach between voluntary and independent sector organisations to come up with a visionary strategic plan to deal with the growing older people population and their increasing demand for care. For them no one agency was in a better position to meet the problems (e.g. P1, 5). It was important at present to review some of the Service Level Agreements with the voluntary sector organisations and delegate some responsibilities to them instead of the family.

> I think what is needed now is for social services and allied agencies such as the health service, the Department for Work and Pensions as well as the voluntary and independent sector organisations to work together... you know... the problem is too big for the families... (P1).

Managers' View

All four managers thought that family care assessors would make an invaluable contribution to reducing waiting time for assessment and care. They asserted that the growing population of older people had left managers with no option but to be proactive and engage all partner agencies to share cost and responsibilities and to plan ahead (e.g. M2, 3). It was argued that family care assessors would help to relieve the pressure on the state, and that social service could work with the family to develop enabling support systems that could enhance social care delivery (M4). Both the Carers Recognition Act and the National Service Framework for older people were referred to as legislative documents that could hopefully help develop a working document to aid collaborative care between social services and the family (M1).

> The state in my opinion cannot cope in meeting the growing care needs of the older people population, without the support of the family... you know. Demand for care is becoming infinite and there is limited supply in the community... My opinion is that we have to somehow rely upon the family... and also to work with them (M4).

Councillors' View

Despite differences in their political opinions, the two councillors shared the same view about reducing waiting times for assessment and care. They thought that engaging the family as care assessors could revolutionise the welfare system for good. This meant that the family should own the responsibility to participate in assessment and provide practical tasks for their older relatives. Social services would only intervene with complex needs or where the cared for person had asked specifically for a social worker, and was prepared for their name to be added to a waiting list. For them, this would be cost effective for the council and the wider community care. Shortage of care workers was a national issue, which could be reduced by involving family members to undertake practical care tasks during care giving.

> You've got an older population growing and growing... we have fewer and fewer carers... I think if we are looking at family members to assess care needs and then be part of the care package, it would help to reduce waiting list for assessment... I do think it would shift responsibilities... (CL1).

> You see... because of medical sciences, probably, the life expectancy is on the increase and social care is becoming complex too. The carers themselves are getting older and in a near future we may find it difficult, you never know... then who would provide care, the government... I don't know... I think family is probably the answer for now maybe... (CL2).

Maintaining Professional Standards
Practitioners' View

Almost all the practitioners (6/7) argued that the family's participation in needs assessment could downgrade professional standards within the welfare service (P5). A proportion of them expressed the view that family members would not be able to carry out a comprehensive assessment as efficiently as professionals. For them family assessment would relegate the role played by the social care workers (e.g. P2, 4, 5). The shift towards family care needs assessment would change the welfare system and social work practice (e.g. 1, 3). It was thought that some of the family caregivers might find it difficult to distinguish between actual needs and potential wants. Some family members also might not be able to ask the right questions during assessment (P6):

> We are suited and capable of doing assessment and implementing it as stated in the Community Care Act. Most social workers apply policy to practice when undertaking needs assessment and that is my professional opinion... Any shift to families... I think would relegate the role played by social workers and that would undermine professional standards (P2).

> We are professionals. We are trained and qualified to carry out social work and care management, some of the family members are not and may find it difficult to distinguish needs, and potential wants... Our aim is to promote and maintain professional standards and professional ethics (P5).

Managers' View

Three of the four managers (3/4) cautioned that any change of emphasis in favour of family caregivers assessing the needs of their older relatives should be gradual and consistent with resource availability and allocation in line with demographic change. Some expressed reservations and said that the approach must be piloted to establish cost implications and benefits to the wider county council (M3, 4). A few made reference to the recent IT software (SWIFT) that was installed within the service. The belief was that the software would enhance recording, storage and retrieval of service users' assessment of needs' data. However, the county council implemented the system without a pilot and that created untold problems with service user's records. Therefore failure to pilot family directed care systems might reduce quality care standards which might not be in the best interests of the service users or their families, or even the wider organisation (M2):

> Family care assessment is a new approach, its potential is yet unknown... it should be piloted otherwise... it would reduce the professional standards and that might not be in the best interest of the service users or their families and the wider organisation (M2).

Councillors' View

Both councillors shared the same view about maintaining professional standards. For them, families undertaking care needs assessment could instigate differences of opinion between the family caregivers and the allocated caseworker (CL1). This could strain their relationship; quality standards and the professionalism of the social workers during care management. Therefore, they would prefer that, the social worker should remain the lead worker with a view to promoting professional standards (CL2). Some care workers might be over-protective of their clients and would not compromise their relationship and professionalism.

> I think sometimes the views and experiences of the family about care and the needs of the older relative's amount to expressions of want rather than needs, and this could damage the professional standards. Some may lack the experience to differentiate needs from want... (CL1).

> Looking at the problems first, I think problems could probably be that a social worker and carer would not agree about the package and about the care needed. There could be

113

very diverse views... you could possibly have a social worker that was overly protective of the service user... they could be very close, and not want too much in the way of family interference so to speak (CL2).

Payment to Family Assessor/Caregiver

The study found divided opinion amongst the three sub-groups. A substantial minority (3/7) of the practitioners, half of the managers (2/4) and one of the two councillors supported the view that the family care assessor or caregiver should be paid. Most argued that it would be cheaper for the council in comparison with the conventional care models of direct provision and direct payments (Chapter s One and Two). In contrast, an almost equal number of the sub-groups (4/7 practitioners, 2/4 managers and ½ councillors) were against the idea and argued that payment to family caregivers would open the floodgates and the council would not be able to afford that. Thematic Dimension Fourteen below represents the views expressed by the sub-groups.

Thematic Dimension 14

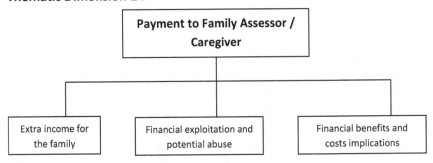

Extra Income for the Family
Practitioners' View

It was argued that family care giving could be influenced by socio-economic factors and family lifestyle. The study showed a significant minority of the practitioners (3/7) supported payment to family caregivers. For some, payment might enhance commitment to continuing care for older relatives (P3). It was argued that payment would help to value and support the roles played by the family caregivers (P4). Payment would mean different things to different people and at the same time it would compensate some for their contribution towards care giving. Family-directed support care systems could take different forms, and the three practitioners argued that payment would be helpful in attracting some family caregivers. Family involvement would help to change the face of the wider welfare service and promote skill mix. That could be an opportunity to expand the social care market (P7).

An extra income for some families could be an attraction to supplement their regular income. People are not at the same level of financial wellbeing; therefore any extra income into the family would act as a reward... I think (P7).

Payment to family care assessor and caregiver was questioned by the majority (4/7). Some argued that it would be unethical for social services to pay family members for offering care to their older relatives. Any payment to family caregivers would challenge the aims and objectives of the welfare service and what it stood for (P1). Some thought that it would open the floodgates and social services would be swamped to pay informal carers for what they were already doing free of charge (P2, 6). Payment to family members for assessment and care would add more pressure on the council's finances, which could affect wider council services (P5). Payment for them is not a panacea to attract family members into the care system rather it is about family's culture, background and reciprocity.

Social services was established as a vocational service and funded by the taxpayers to support all vulnerable users, irrespective of gender, affluence and ageing. Any payment to family carers would change aims and objectives... (P1).

I think it's wrong to pay informal carers for what they are already doing for nothing. I don't think social services would cope, that could put the budget under severe stain (P2)

Managers' View

Two of the four managers (2/4) expressed the view that payment to the family caregiver had the potential to encourage as many of them as possible to commit their limited time towards caring for their older relatives. The extra income would give a great deal of assistance to some family caregivers, which could relieve them of financial burden and stress (M3). They stated that adequate financial support would reduce increasing demand upon them to look for a second job in order to support their nuclear/reconstituted families. Families with an adequate income could hopefully organise themselves within their family system to meet the increasing needs of their older relative and enable them to commit more of their time and effort to care giving (M2).

Payment to the family caregivers would reduce increasing demand upon themselves to rush out to look for second job, for extra income to be able to support their nuclear family and continue care giving their older relatives (M3).

The other two managers (2/4) did not welcome payment to the family caregivers and assessors. They argued that it was against the spirit of socialism and universalism of care giving to older people. One of the managers pointed that the welfare system was created and built up as a vocational service, supported by informal carers and volunteers; otherwise, the state would not be able to sponsor the welfare service. Therefore, any form of payment to families was not supported, because payment would undermine the background history of the service (M4). Although they acknowledged there would be some benefits and contributions that the extra income would make for some families, they felt that a financial incentive was wrong (M1).

Historically the welfare system was created and built as a vocational service, supported by informal care system and volunteers; otherwise, the state would not be able to sponsor the service (M4).

I strongly believe that financial incentive to families is wrong. What is needed within the welfare service is a robust support system such as day care and respite care... that would help families rally round and continue caring for their older relatives (M1).

Councillors' View

The two councillors differed in their views. One of the councillors thought that payment to family caregivers or assessors was a tool that could enhance remodelling of existing practice to suit new demands and the aspirations of older people and the wider welfare system. It was about innovation and creativity linked with modernity. It was also about a shift of care emphasis, away from the state to the family with a view to maximising the family's potential. This would bring about new ideas and different approaches to the delivery of social care for older people in their own home. He reflected that this theme would put the family and the social services on equal levels of understanding of care giving for older relatives.

I think it's about new emphasis and different ways of doing things and meeting older people's needs. That's what I call innovation... I think. Therefore any extra income to the family would act as an inducement to many... those within lower socio-economic classes (CL1).

The other councillor expressed the view that informal carers saved the state a huge sum of money every year. Therefore, any payment to them for care giving was unacceptable. Payment to the families for care giving could ignite conflict or disagreement between the caregiver and the older relative or between the siblings, and that could hinder continuity of care. This probably would be to the disadvantage of the older relatives and as a result payment would not be desirable. She acknowledged that payment might represent an extra income for some families, but cautioned about the ramifications for all concerned.

The problem with family infighting, which you get, and that could create a problem because some of the carers saying, sorry I'm not doing that... because you have been paid to do so and so... no the family should not be paid (CL2).

Financial Exploitation and Potential Abuse
Practitioners' View

A significant majority of the practitioners (5/7) thought that family care giving, to some extent, could encourage financial abuse and this could upset family relationships (P4). Some family caregivers and assessors could exaggerate care packages in order to be paid more money for care giving (e.g. P2, 3, 5). It was thought that there should be a boundary between the family and care giving to older relatives in order to avoid abusive situations and financial misappropriation. Some pointed out that monitoring family care giving would be difficult and expensive for social services because some families were very close and would not disclose any family wrong doing to strangers (e.g. P1, 6, 7):

I feel that this is not a good way forward because, relatives always think there is a greater need than we would assess them for and I doubt if we would be able to afford the needs that the relatives actually assess them for because as I have found, they always assess 200% more than we would do so... this would be very exploitative (P1).

Managers' View

Three of the four managers concluded that payment to the family caregivers or assessors could potentially be an open invitation to financial exploitation and abuse. One thought that financial abuse or exploitation

117

could be difficult to prove (M4). The process of looking into this problem, in line with the No Secret Act (DH 2000), could cost social services and the police dearly in terms of manpower, time and the stress of dealing with any allegations of abuse (M1). The time it would take to deal with this problem by social workers could be invested into assessment and care, making sure that the older relative and their family are supported with their holistic care needs (M3). Most cautioned that a shift in social policy towards family care giving should be thoroughly thought through, making sure that older relatives as well as social services were not exposed to manipulation (M2).

My experience is that moreover where a family is concerned, alleged financial abuse or exploitation sometimes could be difficult to prove. To try to prove that under protection of vulnerable adult (POVA) would cost social services and police a lot of their time, with increased stress of dealing with it (M1).

Councillors' View

Both councillors shared the same view as the other stakeholders. They warned that payment to the family care assessors/caregivers could attract family members who might intend to financially abuse their older relatives and would not provide care. Therefore, a proper vetting system would have to be in place before any agreement was sanctioned by the council (CL2). This would help to reduce the incidence of potential financial abuse or exploitation, which could affect the care continuum within the family care system. The councillors echoed some of the views the other stakeholders expressed regarding the Safeguard of Vulnerable Adults (SOVA) investigations, the stress to the cared for person, and the social workers who might be involved in the care management and investigations.

In practice we have seen it before... some family members caring for their older relative has the potential to financially abuse them or exploiting their vulnerable older relatives... you know (CL1).

Payment I believe would attract all sorts of family members with different characters and this will present some challenges to the council to deal with (CL1).

Financial Benefits and Costs Implication
Practitioners' View

A significant minority of the practitioners (3/7) thought, payment to family caregivers or assessors would not open the floodgates for families to rush to become caregivers overnight (P7). A proportion of them compared family care giving with the direct payments scheme and said it would take a while for the family care giving approach to be embedded into older people's services (P4, P7). Families would take their time to examine and re-examine the advantages and disadvantages of payment to family care assessors and caregivers, before deciding on what to do next (P4). It was thought that family care giving could be cheaper for social services in the long run, rather than the conventional care model of direct provision or direct payments (P1):

> It would definitely be cheaper. The block provider rate now is about £13.95 an hour... so you are talking big differences if we at least pay £8... I think there are limited numbers of people that would be willing, so I don't thin we would flood the market... (P4).

However, the majority (4/7) of the practitioners thought that payment to the family caregivers or assessors could open the floodgates and social services would not be in a position to meet the demand (e.g. P1, 3). Family care giving would not provide a safety net for all of the growing numbers of older people and their needs. It was argued that social services should continue to be the main source of care giving to older people (P5). Some stressed that it was a duty that could not be shifted back to the family, and there were tendencies that family care giving would potentially contribute to an increase in abusive situations and care breakdown (P2). If at all, cost benefits and savings for the council would be minimal, therefore it is worthless pursuing the change/vision.

> The problem here is that family care giving will open the floodgates. Given the present budgetary constraints within the department, social services would not be able to cope with paying family members for what they are already doing free of charge. (P1).

Managers' View

The managers were aware of the relationships between caseworkers' increasing workload and complaints from families and cared for persons during care giving (M3). Some argued that family care giving would help to address these problems and social care workers would be able to concentrate on more demanding tasks within older people's services. They overwhelmingly (4/4) viewed the family care giving approach as complementary and as having the capacity to reduce the overall workload for both the social workers and care providers (e.g. M1, 4). Some pointed out that social care workers would focus and concentrate on more specialist tasks, while the family care assessors/caregivers would undertake non-complex social care tasks. The care model would be an opportunity for specialisation and division of labour within the service (e.g. M1, 3). A few acknowledged that reduced workload as well as specialisation would save a lot of money for the council.

> In my opinion social caseworkers would not be rushing about to attend emergency assessment and care if the family members would take on that responsibility. That would save us more time and money if families were doing such routine tasks. Our time could be used more cost effectively... (M4).

Councillors' View

Consistent with the previous findings, one of the councillors thought family care assessors or caregivers would help the council to save some money. He welcomed family care assessment and care giving that would enhance the financial standing of the council, because the care model might help to reduce the number of complaints that social workers had to deal with on a daily basis. He affirmed that social care workers' workload had increased to an extent, because of families' complaints about poor quality of care giving. He explained that if the family were providing the care, then there would be a tendency that complaints would be reduced to a minimum:

> Yes, I think it probably would, because possibly the relatives would themselves see some of the problems at first hand... often the complaints you get are probably from a relative who doesn't have regular contact, and they will go away and come back... don't see them for a week or two weeks, and they come back, why is that not happening, why has that happened...? (CL1).

On the contrary, the councillor from the Left argued that family care assessment or care giving would not save any money for the council. She cited most of the potential problems highlighted above (lack of knowledge of assessment and care giving, compliance with regulations, relegation of professional standards and poor quality of care) as issues of concern to the image of social services and to its budget. She argued that what was needed was for the family to continue as informal carers. Social workers would assist them with accurate and adequate information and signpost them to appropriate resource centres that would help them to continue care giving. She stated that information and advice were central to the effective support systems available within social services and other welfare organisations (CL2):

> The council would not allow itself to be criticised because of negligence propagated by the family's inconsistent approach to offer assistance and care to their older relatives. The implications to the council are that it would cost more money to remedy such mistakes made by the family caregivers/assessors. Family care giving might lead to what I call economic waste... (CL2).

Conclusion

Focusing on emotional needs themes, the study overall found that a significant minority (3/7) of the practitioners, half of the managers (2/4) and one of the two councillors thought that family care giving was well placed to provide emotional care for their older relatives in comparison with strangers. On the other hand, over one half (4/7) of the practitioners, half of the managers (2/4) and the other councillor expressed concerns. Most cited the critical and substantial nature of the current social services eligibility criteria matrix as an issue of concern. Despite some of the misgivings expressed by some of the sub-groups' members, 5/7 practitioners, 3/4 managers and one councillor affirmed that knowing the caregiver would promote stability and participation during care giving. Most of the three sub-groups – 5/7 practitioners, 3/4 managers and one councillor – expressed some reservation about family care needs assessment and care giving. Most thought that social workers were better positioned to carry out a comprehensive and efficient care needs assessment. However, it is important to note that the majority of the sub-groups – 4/7 practitioners, 3/4 managers and one councillor – acknowledged that family care giving could reduce waiting times between assessment and care. Consistent with the findings, the sub-groups were divided in their opinions. Over one half (4/7) of the practitioners, one half of the managers (2/4) and one of the councillors were against payment to family caregivers and assessors. In contrast, a considerable minority of practitioners (3/7), two of the four managers and one of the councillors supported the view that payment to family caregivers would not open the floodgates.

Chapter Five:
Sustainability of Personalisation

Introduction

Older people valued personal social services highly and had clear views about what characterises quality in these services. Practice observations conclude that older people are now articulated and wish to take control of their later life care with adequate support systems. As the baby boomers are entering the care systems, they are able to dictate the qualities they deserved as part of their home care packages that could sustain their needs in the community. A number of research have outlined the basic and essential qualities and what older people want with regard to their later life care (Patmore 2002, 2003, 2005; Raynes et al 2001, 2005; Joseph Rowntree Foundation 2009).

Care in a Challenging Democracy

Clearly, the current macro and micro-economic situations within the economy have been particularly challenging for the social care market, with considerable political paradigm shift and the severe budget deficit in the UK. The challenges now is not just ensuring health and social care are delivered to an even better standard, but to ensure this is done with considerably fewer resources. Now, more than ever, it is vital that it is clearly understood who and what needs to be in place in the future to guarantee effective and efficient delivery of health and social care to older people.

The vision for sustainability of later life care are to uphold a holistic assessment of functional activities of daily living; taking adequate care to risk identifications and management. Offering older people choice and control would promote personalisation and sustainability of independent living and participation in their care. These perspectives among other things; enhances psycho-social wellbeing as well as assisting older people to determine their own social care solutions. Intuitionally, assessment and review of care is a key to sustainability whilst, decision making for enabling support systems clearly define the objectives of care and overreaching outcomes being sought henceforth.

Personalisation of services has provided the platform for older people if able to access *"individualised budget, cash for care or direct payments"* in anyway that could meet their assessed needs. Their preference to a care model would illuminate best value, and marketisation of social care hence these provide the opportunity for the service to be within budget and accountable. Sustainability however, brings about effectiveness of delivering social care to older people; efficient management of limited resources whilst delivering quality of care and a vision for economic and proactive sourcing and procurement of services. These dimensions are interrelated to achieving person centred service i.e. providing care that meets individual needs, taking into account risk management and all functional activities of daily living at no extra cost.

Reformulated, individual programme plan (IPP) would give older people and their caregiver's real and informed choice to determine their wellbeing and be free from potential abuse and discrimination in the service. Older people and their carers stand to work together and utilise social workers' knowledge and expertise in conjunction with other professional agencies such as the healthcare workers. Collaboration in this instant would create a lasting opportunities to resolve problems of co-ordination and just in time care management approach. Thus, all the key stakeholders have the propensity to work together with the aim to dissolve hierarchical management structures between health and social care, with the hope to achieve sustainability in the services delivery.

New Challenges to Professional Health and Social Care Workers

The new coalition government is intended to overhaul health and social care sector in order to maximize its aims to balance the nation's budget. The aim is to scrutinize and the impact of the two distinctive to some extent and interrelated ideological positions of New Labour and the coalition government of the Conservative and the Liberal Democrat' parties.The question is what impact would this have on health and social care professionals and the delivery of services to older people and their families.

Health and social care sector have seen avalanche of changes in the last thirty years for example, the NHS and Community Care Act (1990), modernization of health and social services (personalization of Services) (DH 2005) and the Big Society (Cameron 2010). These policy frameworks tend to formalise assessment of health and social care needs, provider/

purchaser split, and cash for care frameworks. The reforms paved the way to identify individualised care packages appropriate to meet service users care needs either in their own home or in a residential care setting. Yet, older people and their informal caregivers have not been adequately served. Their plight have been highlighted by a number of authorities such as Twigg and Atkin (1994), Carers National Association (2001), Help the Aged (2002), Lewis (2004, 2006), Carers Act (2007) and Glendinning et al (2008).

The question is would the "Big Society" replicate the "Third Way" approach or in what way would it deliver effective and adequate health and social care for older people. All these perspectives talks about partnership working between the state and users, collaboration of services between agencies, empowerment, choice and control. New Labour attempted to represent a new social democratic order – a different approach to government, in which, the state should not dominate, but steer not so much control to deliver public services. The "Big Society" is about liberation – the biggest, most dramatic redistribution of power from the government and state to the man and woman on the street (Cameron 2010). However, would the policy framework present difficulties for professionals to deliver health and social care to older people and informal caregivers? It is too early to express concerns, yet it is imperative to mention the potential risks, which could be present whilst pursuing the "Big Society" agenda. Thus, risk is defined as; the uncertainty of outcome, whether positive opportunity or negative threat, of actions and events. The risk has to be assessed in respect of the combination of the likelihood of something happening, and the impact, which arises if it does actually happen. The Big Society is relatively unknown at present, but the practical initiatives are for the professionals to understand the type of potential risks that are likely to present difficulties to deliver health and social in the present climate.

Type of potential Risks and challenges

- Risk to service users, which may include safeguarding of vulnerable adults (SOVA). Abuse includes: Physical, Sexual, Negligence, Financial and Deprivation (DoH 2000)
- Risk to paid carers, who may be employed by the local authority or independent section organizations or private.
- Risk to the public, the individual concern, family members or the carers.
- Risk to Infrastructure or organizational, that arising from service or facilities issue, including third party providers or partners.

- Environmental risk such as sever weather, public health or pollution issues subject to emergency planning.

- Legal and Regulatory risks such as the legality of items in a support plan or compliance with legislation.

- Reputational risks, which could affect the public or the government reputation.

- Financial and budgetary risks arising from the availability and allocation of resources, fraud or theft.

Reasonable risk

Reasonable risk is about striking a balance between empowering people to make choices, while supporting them to take informed everyday risk. Thus, the aim of this policy is to create a sound framework for professional judgment and adequate decision making in relation to the management of either the actual risks or the potential risks and to support those involved to explore the issues and make arrangements which go as possible towards meeting the individual service users aspirations, whilst balancing the needs and risks to themselves. Risk management is an important and necessary process that enables the professionals to maximize opportunities and creativity in every day operations as well as identifying threats to the service. This is in line with "Putting People First", a shared vision and commitment to the transformation and personalization of services (Care Services Improvements Partnerships 2007; CSCI 2006a). Risk identifications and management would provide the opportunity to deliver personalised social care to older people hence their wish is to remain in their own home for as long as possible. Home support services are enhanced by adherence of the concepts outlined below and these would provide assurance to older people that their needs are met bearing in mind their lifestyles.

Home Support Services
Carers Activities

Older people want to be aware of any changes in carers or carers' activities so that they will not open their doors to strangers. They want carers to be trained in the tasks they have to do and trained to listen to clients. Older people should be notified of tasks they could expect carers to undertake. However, some older people currently have no way of knowing what their carer can do for them. Knowing this would remove some uncertainty for them. According to Twigg (2006) and Carers National Association (2001), there seems to be little opportunity to negotiate changes needed in the help older people want as their needs change. Older people felt a quality service would ensure that a list of tasks that can be done by home carers is provided annually and those carers are flexible enough to address particular short-term needs and reflect longer-term changes in the help that is needed.

Aids and Equipment

Aids and Equipment is important to sustain both independence and inter-dependence with family caregiver as this have been contended by previous studies such as Raynes et al (2001) and Joseph Rowntree Foundation (2007, 2009). Older people highly valued aids and adaptations of all kinds in their home as these would help to promote independence for as long as possible in the community. This would mean a service that could enable them to regain some of their independence in or outside their home. Practice observations indicated that provision of essential aids such as grab rails, walking frames, walk-in showers, seats in showers, stair lifts; panic and pendant alarms would provide them the comfort they deserve without relying solely on their carers. Getting out of their home could be difficult for some older people without assistance of aids/equipment of some sort such as walking stick or wheelchair. Having helped to get away from their house was seen as an important attribute of a quality home care service. Some of these support systems have long waiting lists and some local authorities do not triage some of the services as priority. The considerable difficulties experienced by older people in accessing services has been highlighted by a number of people as well as in reports such as Carers National Association (2001), Help the Aged (2002) and Lewis (2005), yet their condition has not been improved within the welfare system.

Transportations

Older people saw good, safe transport and better health care services as essential part of social care services. Both services promoted independence and affected their attitudes to their lives in their own homes. Neither transport nor health care is currently defined as social care services. However, older people saw these services as complementary support systems to an enhanced social care. Both Lewis and Surender (2004) and Joseph Rowntree Foundation (2009) noted that older people valued accessible and affordable transport, designed so that they could get out and back to their homes safely without being physically distressed. According to King's Fund (2006), older people indicated that health care services such as regular check-ups by their GPs and regular review of their repeat prescriptions contributed to the quality health and social care services. However, some of these services are not available in some localities, making it difficult for some older people to remain in their home for as long as possible (Commission for Social Care Inspectorate 2007).

Telecare Systems

Successful home care and assisted living for older people is depended upon a holistic assessment framework carried out by assessors who are able to identify risks and draw up strategic risk management plans to overcome the risks within their surrounding environment. The Social Work Task Force Board identified among other things: the need for more emphasis on risk assessment frameworks; risk analysis and joint working with other professionals such as the occupational therapists. Telecare systems are changing the face of home care for older people within the wider welfare services. Telecare by definition is electronic tools (sensor mat, medication alert system, task alert reminder) designed and capable to assisted living in the community. These devices are now helping many older people to achieve their aspirations and to be cared for in their own home. Most local authorities prefer to maintain, as many older people as possible in the community rather than in residential care settings and telecare have been instrumental to achieve this policy framework. The systems also provide assurance to some family members that their older relatives are safe in their own home and potential risks are reduced. To greater extent, telecare has enhanced home life environment, older people are no longer compelled to move into residential home setting because of risks within their environment. Here are some examples of Telecare systems that have enhanced end of life care and it has boosted older people's confidence to be cared in their own home rather than placing them in a residential or nursing care home settings:

1. **MemRabel:** is a stylish timepiece developed to assist people with dementia, learning disabilities and people with cognitive problems live a more independent life. To associate time in relation to daylight and night time hours, the clock displays daylight hours with an icon of the sun and an icon of the moon for night time hours. MemRabel can be used as a daily time clock, alarm clock and voice memory aid/reminder. It also has features that aid care of people with the above conditions to provide warnings and alarms. It has four alarm time reminders with the option to record a different voice memo for each alarm. The message is played back at alarm time. The duration of the repeated alarm playback can be set for 3, 6, or 9 minutes. Alarms can be set for

hourly, daily or weekly playback. Memos can be used to remind of tasks, medicine reminders or instructions

2. ***The SAT-01:*** is a useful sound monitoring product that produces an alarm signal to a selected level of sound. The product can be used to listen out for people that may require help but are unable to press a button, of a nurse call system for example. It is suitable for use in the home or for professional care and is available with a choice of paging options to suit your alarm/alert requirements. For monitoring a single patient and the product is ideal as the pager produces a strong vibration with optional levels of alarm sounds The SAT-01 is mains powered via DC power adaptor and has 36 hour battery backup provides by a built in rechargeable battery. Controls of the SAT-01 are very simple with just a sensitivity control for the microphone level. A detect LED lights to indicate detected sounds.

3. ***Bed/chair Sensor:*** bed or chair leaving sensors with alarm pager for people at risk from falls and is for home use or institutional care home/hospital If you need an alarm to detect a person leaving their bed or chair the equipment detailed on this page will provide a reliable, economical solution. The system comprises of a sensor mat, bed or chair, a wireless monitor transmitter and a radio pager. For a bed, the sensor is placed under the patents mattress of bed sheet, for a chair under the chair cushion or seat cover. When the patient sits or lies down, the monitor transmitter acknowledges detection with a couple of beeps. When the patient rises an alarm signal is transmitted to the radio pager, which can be up to 150M away. Either system can be set up in a couple of minutes. The new extended alarm delay option can be selected to allow the user 15 minutes to go to the bathroom etc before the alarm signal is transmitted to the alarm pager.

4. ***The Medpage MP-6:*** uses the same technology as the MP5 to detect convulsive nocturnal seizures. The equipment is supplied with 2 x care giver pagers (one as a backup) that produce variable volume alarm tones with vibration or vibration only. The equipment latch on when a seizure is detected. An LED stays lit and a built in low volume buzzer operates until the alarm is manually reset by pressing the red reset button. The product is equipped with a single bed sensor that is positioned in-between the bed base and bed mattress. A control is provided to fine tune

sensitivity of the sensor to the user and type of bed they sleep in. A delay control provides delay on alarm to help minimise false alarms. Normal movements such as turning over or coughing will not cause an alarm. The product has battery backup providing in excess of 72 hours operation on backup power. .Setup of the alarm is very simple as there is a movement detect LED that lights when the sensor control is correctly set. The MP6 will send an alarm signal by radio transmitter to the alarm pagers at distances of up to 100 Metres (line of sight). In a building 50 Metres would be expected depending on the construction of the building. It is equipped with an output socket that can be used to directly connect the monitor into a nurse call system or to a telephone auto dialler for people with Epilepsy that live alone and wish to have a remote alarm to contact relatives, friends or neighbours who can help them when a seizure is ongoing. The output socket can also be connected to a data logger to capture seizure activity and times

5. ***Automatic fall alarm with telephone auto dialler the standard fall alarm system (FAS-1)*** consists of a fall detector, worn like a pager by the user and a telephone auto dialler. The fall detector has a belt clip for attachment to a belt or clothing and is equipped with a simple on-off switch. When the detector is switched on, any sudden movement or tilt from a vertical to a horizontal position will result in a pre-alarm tone that will sound for 30 seconds prior to transmitting the emergency control signal to activate the telephone dialler. This provides sufficient time for the user to cancel the alarm to avoid false dialling to the recipients on the call list. The telephone dialler can store up to six of your own emergency contact telephone numbers. When the dialler receives a signal from the fall alarm, the automatic dialling sequence begins. The first number will be called. If the call is answered the dialler will announce emergency then speak your home telephone number. If the first call recipient can attend to the emergency, they can use their telephone keypad to cancel all further calls on the call list. If they are unable to deal with the incident, they can simply hang up leaving the dialler to call the next number on the call list and so on until calls are cancelled by disarming the dialler using the keypad or by a call recipient telephone. If the call is answered by a mobile telephone voicemail, or a land line answer machine, the message will be left. The dialler will then go on to dial the

remaining numbers on your call list (http://www.tunstall.co.uk/
Our-products/Telecare-solutions/Individual-homes).

Institutional care is an environment where, despite good intentions, there is a great imbalance of power between the residents and those providing care or support them. This power imbalance can also arise when older people receive a lot of support at home. From practice based observation, it could be argued that low self-esteem amongst older people living in different kinds of supported accommodation (residential care home' sheltered accommodation) is a huge and multifaceted issue. Low expectations of a fulfilling life are issues of concern and as a result older people prefer to remain and receive care in their own home for as long as possible. Research such as Raynes et al (2001, 05) indicated that older people rejected institutional care in favour of home care because there is a clear lack of strong and unifying vision of good life for older people with high support needs. Increasing choice for older people and their carers or families has been one of the cornerstones of government policy, both Conservative and New Labour. The NHS and Community Care Act (DoH 1990), and more recently the Royal Commission on Long-Term Care for Older People (1999), aimed to ensure that older people have increased opportunities to stay at home rather than enter residential care. Jospeh Rowntree (2009) argued that this was the choice of older people and their carers/families, and that more resources should be put into enabling them to satisfy that choice. Telecare systems should form a significant part of home care package for older people and their informal caregivers, which could significantly ease longevity of care.

Tapping Family Potential

Historically, family care giving has played a dominant role in caring for the older and younger members of the family in our society. This view has been supported by previous studies such as Phillipson et al (2001), Haslar (2002) and Lewis (2002, 2004, 2006). This experience revealed that many older people and their families are of the view that family caregivers have the potential to offer more emotional and practical care for their older relatives during end of life care, rather than strangers. Some of their reasons are fear of strangers; knowing the person providing care; sharing family norms and values as well as fulfilling duties and responsibilities. Intuitively, family care system would be more appropriate than conventional service frameworks such as direct provision, direct payments or cash for care. Given that people (85+) are living longer, frail and disabled, they would be incapacitated to manage their own care

(Sale and Leason 2004; Bredaet al 2006). In most cases older people and their family caregivers value enabling support systems such as aids and equipment, respite and day care, shared care packages. Support for family caregivers would encourage them immensely to continue care giving to their older relatives. Aids and equipment would reduce dependency levels, accidents, falls and potential deterioration in health amongst the family caregivers and the cared for person. Day and respite care would enable carers to have breaks from care and recuperate from continuing care to their older relatives (Secker et al 2003).

> I've got a walking frame and I get about walking like that but I've got to have a bag to put on it to carry things in and out and my daughter, she goes to work from about 9 a.m. until about 4 p.m., see... five days a week, she works for herself, so I've got the access to the front room.

Reflecting on assessment for later life care, practice observation suggest that older people and the family caregivers thought that families are best placed to carry out needs assessment rather than social workers. Family members know the cared for person and their needs better, and would be able to draw up a flexible care plan that would accommodate a holistic need for their older relatives during the period of care giving (Finch 1998; Wilkinson 2000). The statement below surmises the view and experience of a service user during care needs assessment:

> You know I've lived with him for a long time. No one knows him better than I do... I will like to carry out his needs assessment and care for him because he can be an actor sometimes... I know my father well and have been caring for him since he became ill and unable to care for himself. I think I can draw up his needs from memory. His needs change every day therefore assessment I think is ongoing depending on his mood.

Personalisation and Reablement for later life enhances is pointing towards "the Big Society" concept and implementation of the ideology within the wider personalisation of social care for older people. This provides the opportunity to manage the ageing population and longevity of care in the 21st Century and beyond. The service framework for older people (DoH 2001) and modernization of health and social care (DoH 2005, 2008) reinvigorates the opportunity for innovation and creativity that are highly needed in social care organisation. This interfaced with the whole systems approach and community wellbeing in line with the "Big Society" agenda of the coalition government of the Conservative and the Liberal Democrat parties.

The "Big Society" policy framework is a wake up call for communities, families and individuals to come together and share the responsibilities for the growing older people's care needs, more over those aged 85 and above. Care and support planning for later life and assisted living for older people is a care model that emphasises the need for social reengineering within families and communities to participate in their older relatives care. History has shown that family's involvement and their supporting activities revolve endlessly (Shana 1948; Phillipson et al 2001).This is aimed to reshape the collective welfare systems and transfers social care responsibilities to the family and the service user to take control of their care needs.This would reduce red tape and bureaucratic systems within care management approach and community care assessment process (DoH 1990).

Social work practice experience and a number of previous studies (Lewis and Meredith 1988; Lewis 2002 and 2004) has shown that older people want to participate in their later life care plan, development and implementations to high standards as they are used to. Personalisation of care and assisted living by family members or community support groups offers older people the opportunity to live for as long as possible in their own home. The "Big Society" rekindles family and community responsibilities, empowerment and participation in decision making about their lives and their long-term care. The Service Framework for Older People (2001) demonstrates the importance of family, individuals and community's commitment, and maximisation of resources within the social care sector. Family and community involvements would promote family commitments, participation and shared responsibilities.

The "Big Society's" vision of care approach would in practice; reduce waste in the system, improves high standards of care and value for money on the long run. It proposes three major shifts in public services policy: Local, community or family members should set up mutual and co-operatives to run public services, including leisure or day centres; there should be a radical shift in power from central government to the most local level. Where possible, citizens should commission services themselves using individual budgets and choice advisors and neighbourhood should control their own integrated services; public finances should be more open, transparent and understandable to citizens, with on line statement of contributions and benefits available to everyone (Cameron 2010). These statements reflected Lewis and Meredith (1988), Wilkinson (1998, 2000), Lewis (2004, 2005, 2007) and Glendinning et al (2009) philosophy and

132

wisdom of family care systems and the benefits to older people and the state.End of care strategy has become a national issue given longevity of care giving to older relatives and delivery of care could be enhanced by good leadership approach within social work authorities.

Leadership in Social Work Practice

Good leadership approach would hernece modernisation and personalisation of services for the vulnerable services users in society. Visonary thinking within professional social work would work in paralle to the delivery of the Big Society agenda. This bearing in mind the constriction of the formal social care workers and the family units.This ideological concept brings to light the issues of poor leadership in social work practice, which lack clear vision in professional social work and changing social care needs of the emerging ageing population. The exploration of the concerns would lead to evolution of the profession and its entire endeavour in the 21st Century and beyond. Visionary leadership would enhance what the author called *"Just in Time Care Management Approach"*.

This perspective coincides with the *"Big Society"* ideology of power to the people, community involvements, and effective resource management at minimum costs.The looming public sector budget cuts will likely result in wide-ranging and potentially radical changes within social services and the rolesplayed by numerous social workers. Many workers feel destabilised by change – even if it does not directly affect them, while others may experience increased stress while doing their job with fewer colleagues or resources. Therefore, the leaders in professional social work should muster dynamic qualities to build teams that are motivated, engaged, confident and efficient even in the face of tough challenges.

One of the key influencers in retaining a stable and motivated team is if those changes come from the top. A good leader is much more than 'just a manager'. A good leader will master four universal leadership goals that are crucial for a cohesive and successful working environment – increasing trust and communication, managing conflict in a professional way, building organisational capability and driving organisational strategy. Leaders who achieve these goals will be better placed to guide teams through any storm. The emphasis within social services and the wider welfare organisations are to help employees or workers understand their own working behaviours. This would enable them to work more effectively as this is something crucial to success with reduced teams. Equally crucial is for leaders to understand their employees' behaviours. Practice experience revealed that a number of workers or employees feel their managers didn't understand their skills, preferences and motivations.

Using accessible psychometric tools to examine and acknowledge what drives social care workers and where their strengths and talents lie is invaluable in making the most of teams, especially as resources tighten. It also helps indentify how professionals respond to change, allowing leaders to recognise and mitigate areas of stress that may escalate to conflict. Any change can make employees feel unsettled, often triggering a drop in motivation and productivity. Rather than bury heads in the sand, it is therefore crucial that employers acknowledge change, and keep staff abreast with developments. The more that staff feel informed about changes being made, and their impact, the quicker they will be able to accept those changes and re-engage with the organisation.

Equally, cutting budgets shouldn't mean cutting important activities like training. Training and development help social care workers feel appreciated and engaged; meaning if their job description has also changed, they will be more able to keep up and keep motivated.During times of change, it is more important than ever to focus on the people in your organisation. There may be pressures to divert attention into simply getting the job done, but the risks of overlooking employees' needs when times are tough, and funds tight, may well outweigh any cost-saving measures being implemented. It's not about having agood leader.If the aim is for the organisation to focus on people as much as money and other resources then what is required is for all managers to show leadership qualities. Managers at every level in the organisation that have the leadership qualities need to be confident enough to explain decisions without appearing defencive or ridged in their views. A good leader is some one who can make subordinates feel valued during usterity meassures that affect all arms of the organisation. A leader strives to create rapport and work with his/her staff to deliver high quality services in increasingly difficult circumstances.

The modern social work needs a strong leadership approach that is able to conceptualise the cross cultural enterprise and care interface between health and social care institutions. Leadership is always a relative process. To be effective and to communicate ideas as intended, a leader would always modify his behaviour to take into account the expectations of all the key stakeholders and interpersonal skills of those with who service users interact with. There can be no specific rules of leadership, which will work well in all situations owing to geo-political influences and other environmental factors. The broad principles such as consultative, democratic and facilitating can be applied in the process of leadership and these should be inculcated in a manner that takes fully into account the challenges of demographic change and the aspirations of the service users.

For leaders to function well; they may have to combine natural intelligence, practice based-knowledge and formal training opportunities to develop a flexible leadership style capable enough to lead subordinates. Social work is now changing with time and challenges from users therefore, the profession has to keep pace with the characteristics of good leadership skills and styles in order to achieve results that are expected by the stakeholders.

Conclusion

Growing older can be a worrying moment in our lives, more over when we know what lies ahead for example, frailty, infirmities, dementia and other related old age diseases. Thus, our hopes and care is then mortgaged in the hands of other people. This can be a horrifying journey for all of us, but the questions are who is best you support you throughout this lonely and terrifying moment. My professional and human instinct suggests that family care systems would prevail. At a macroeconomic level, the welfare systems are overstretched and unable to carter for the social care needs of the growing older people population and their increasing demand for care needs. The public sector spending is said to crowd out the private sector. At corporate level, the expanding state is presumed to stifle entrepreneurs with taxes and regulations. At individual level, welfare payments are said to foster dependency and discourage ambition. At informal family care levels, family and cultural enterprise is not fostered and supported fully. In this regards who is best to sustain the best interest of the emerging older people population, moreover if the anticipated public spending is cut to the bones.

Chapter Six:
Personalisation beyond Informal Care Giving

Introduction

The thrust of personalisation and reciprocal family care giving theory is that the decline in family care giving is the result of the deterioration of older relatives' status and role, as a consequence of the breakdown of the traditional extended family and the emergence of isolated nuclear and socio-economic influences. As a result, the increased emphasis on the primacy of the bonds between spouses and their dependent children, older relatives become trapped in a "role-less role" with children or relatives no longer ready or prepared to pay them much attention or support (Burgess 1960; Townsend 1968; Phillpson et al 2001). Ultimately, declining family care giving is being seen as caused by increasing physical strains, financial difficulties of both the cared for person and their families, burden of care giving and to an extent the unwillingness of the adult children or kin to provide care for their older relatives. This chapter is narrated within three sub-themes: the explanatory content of the family care giving; psychological perspective to personalisation and reciprocal family care giving; the exploration of personalisation and reciprocal family care giving.

The Explanatory Content of the Family Care Giving

This explanation was advanced to clarify the socio-economic difficulties that most would be family caregivers face and which have caused widespread poverty amongst them (Wilkinson 1998, 2000; Help the Aged 2002). It is much more likely because of smaller family unit, geographical mobility since the 1950s, women's work outside the home, and the expectation that the welfare state would provide adequate services, for which we all pay for during our working lives (Machin et al

1994; Pickard et al 2000; Lewis 2004). Declining family care giving was highlighted in the United Nations (1999), who set up new international plans of action on ageing. The plans were ratified at the second World Assembly on Ageing in April 2002 and were intended as a blueprint for policy formulation in member States:

> Migration, urbanisation, the shift from extended to smaller, mobile families and other socio-economic changes can marginalise older people, taking away their purposeful economic and social roles and weakening their traditional source of support (UN 2002:9).

Despite its importance, personalisation of services and reciprocal family care giving theory's explanations for actual shifts or inadequacies in the family care giving and payment to family caregivers, have received much less empirical or theoretical attention in the UK and other European countries, this is despite acknowledgment of the importance of informal care giving as an integral part of a mixed economy of care in the community (Twigg and Atkin 1994; King's Fund 2006; Joseph Rowntree Foundation 2009; Glendinning et al 2009). Thus, the growing older people population and their increasing care needs have indicated the need for rethinking social policy for older people and the wider welfare systems.

Demographic Change

The falling childbirth rate leads to fewer younger people in the population and hence a rise in proportion of older peoples (Office for National Statistics 2001; O'Hara 2004). The total childbirth rate within the UK was 5% at the end of the 19th century. This decreased to a lower rate of 1.7% in 1933 and rose again during the post-war baby boom to 2.8 % in 1947. It reached an increased rate during the baby boom of the 1960s of 3% in 1964 but has continued to decrease steadily ever since to the current rate of 1.7% (Evandrou 1998). Ageing population is not just a UK problem but a global trend (United Nations organisation 1982, 99, 02).

Most countries in the Western world are experiencing a significant drop in childbirth and an increasing ageing population which has resulted in a dramatic decrease in the working population, mostly in the health and social care industry (O'Hara 2004). Europe is one of the continents with a high number of older people who require a high level of care giving (Organisation for Economic Co-operation and Development 1998 a & b; Ruddock et al 1998). Some European countries have experienced low childbirth since the 1970s, leading to a higher proportion of the population being aged 65 and over. This is because the childbirth rate is lower in these countries, and many have sustained low birth levels over a long period of time (Kinsella and Velkoff 2001). The implication of the falling birth rate means that the increasing care needs of older people will continue to be a problem for social services, the families and the older people themselves.

Ageing population and falling birth rate have social and financial implications for both social services and families leading to considerable interest in the future care needs of older relatives and availability of reciprocal family care giving. Although the need for carers was explicitly recognised in the Department of Health (1995, 2000a), it remains unclear what impact these reforms have had on informal carers. As Rowland (1998) noted, the intention of those reforms was to address inadequate service provision and support to carers. However, Carers National Association (2001) argued that the level of support for informal carers had declined in recent times. It is now widely known that for the next twenty to thirty years the demographic characteristics of the population will continue to undergo rapid and increasing. The age profile is seeing a major growth in those aged 65+, and this is more marked amongst the 85+ groups of whom many are even carers to their spouses. Ruddock et al (1998) argued that the combination of these factors could potentially affect the physical health and psychosocial well-being of some family caregivers in the long run. Thus, implementation of family directed support care systems as a dynamic option for service framework within the wider welfare systems would help to promote personalised care delivery for older people.

Family Carers in Policy Discourse

This section considers first at the ways in which carers are viewed in policy terms then at what has been put in place or suggested by way of support. The Carers National Association (2001) claimed that family caregivers are not only involved in providing personal, psychological and emotional care, but are also providing highly intensive and technical care for their relatives. This growing concern was in part fuelled by the feminist critique that emphasised the exploitative character of community care and that exposed the compulsory self-sacrifice that underlay it (Ungerson 1987; Dalley 1998). As a result, the needs of carers are increasingly featured on the policy agenda: politicians of different persuasions have expressed concerns about carers' welfare and the need to support them to carry out their role in the wider welfare systems – Carers (Recognition and Services) Act (DoH 1995) and Carers and Disabled Children Act – DoH 2000).

However, the growing emphasis on the needs of carers has been criticised within the disability groups. Disabled people are asserting their rights to independence and claimed that support to carers simply under-writes a dependency culture (Oliver 1990; Morris 1991). Within the welfare systems, family caregivers occupy on the one hand a strategic position and on the other, their position seems ambiguous within the care system and this makes it hard to establish the relationship between carers and public agencies.The various Carers legislation as stated above has played a major role in defining who the carer is, yet there remains some ambiguity in the policy framework in terms of carers' roles and how they are supported. However, Twigg (1992) and Twigg and Atkin (1993, 94) have conceptualised these ambiguities in four models of how public agencies related to family caregivers:

Carers as Resources

In practice, family caregivers represent the reality of community care and a large proportion of caregivers to older people with frailty and disabilities are from the informal sector – possibly family members. Twigg and Atkins argued that informal caregivers represent the "taken-for-granted" reality against which agencies operate. Informal caregivers or family members are regarded as coming first, with the assumption that services need only step in when it is unavailable. Carers are featured only as part of the background, and the agency is largely unconcerned with carers' welfare. The agencies' concern is to maximise care; and there is often a fear that the formal services will take the place of informal care Twigg and Atkin 1994).

Carers as Co-workers

Family directed support care system demonstrates the opportunity to work alongside the informal caregiver or family member, intertwining agency support with that of the caregiver. In most cases in practice, family caregivers or informal caregivers are seen as co-workers in a joint care packages or double handed case.Twigg (1993, 2006) contends that the primary focus for agencies is still on the service user, but in a way that recognises the importance of the morale of the carer, both for continuance of care and for its quality. The co-worker model encompasses the caregiver's interest and well-being amongst its concerns, but on an essentially instrumental basis. Conflict of interests are recognised, but seen as something that could be resolved.

Carers as Co-clients

In this context, informal caregivers are regarded as people in need of support in their own right. Support systems are aimed at helping them with their care needs and also promoting their independence. Both

Twigg (2006) and Twigg and Atkin (1993, 94) claimed that the use of the term "carers" is limited, confined only to those cases where the informal caregivers are heavily burdened or stressed. The focus of intervention is the caregiver and his/her welfare is also considered. The conflict of interest is fully recognised, though the primary emphasis is placed on the problems this poses for the carer.

Superseded Carers

The aim is not to draw on or support the care giving relationship, but to go beyond or supersede it. Twigg and Atkin (1993, 94) suggested two avenues to achieve this model. The first measure is to try to maximise the service user's independence. The aim is not to ease the lot of carers, but to free service users from a relationship of dependence with their caregivers. The second route comes from a concern with the carers. Maximising the independence of the service user will potentially do away with the need for carers and with it the burdens of care giving. The focus of intervention is either on the caregiver or the cared for person depending on which route has been a priority. Either way the caregiver or the cared for person are seen as separate beings. Conflict of interest is fully recognised, and from the viewpoint of both and the valued outcome is independence for both.

Carers Support

Government policy over the last twenty years has been to support informal carers. The Health and Social Care Act (DoH 2001), the Carers and Disabled Children Act (DoH 2000) and Carers (Recognition and Services) Act (DoH 1995), noted that carers have needed that support in order to continue care giving for their older relatives. The National Carers Strategy (DoH 1999a) represents the most ambitious attempt yet to support informal carers in their caring role. The National Service Framework for Older People emphasised the need to support carers and to establish systems to explore users' and carers' experiences in care giving roles (Department of Social Security 1998b; DoH 2000, 2001a).Research evidence (Carers National Association 2001; Help the Aged 2002) indicated that caregivers needed this support. A carer's own health may be adversely affected, while many caregivers were ageing and finding it increasingly difficult to continue care giving. However, with the current absence of adequate training and information available to carers, this would mean a reduction in the number of family caregivers willing to offer their support to older relatives. Despite these concerns, the White Paper Modernising Social Care (DoH 1998a, 2000, 2001) contained no identifiable fresh sources of support for carers. Johnson (1987) made two points about the role of the informal caregivers.

Firstly, it is unlikely that it can compensate for any reduction in statutory services for older people. Social and demographic changes are reducing the capacity for family care giving, at a time when the number requiring care is increasing. Secondly, if the purpose of welfare pluralism is to extend choice, then it should not be geared to pressurising people into taking on extra responsibilities. In cases where people choose to care for dependent relatives, they should be given information and advice about the relevant services available to them in the community as well as any existing services (Johnson 1987).

Psychological Perspectives to Personalisation and Reciprocal Family Care

The core values of personalisation and reciprocal family care giving can be clearly defined as: respect for individuals' dignity, striving to provide a family orientated support system that promotes autonomy, confidentiality, choice that re-establishes family reciprocity; and social re-engineering within the family. One of the advantages of personalisation of services and family care giving is that some families have common identity, values and attitudes which they share and that form the rules that guide social behaviour within the family cohesion (Lewis and Meredith 1988; Wilkinson 2000; Lewis 2004).

Family advocacy and participation in care giving for older relatives is seen as a vehicle for promoting social behaviour which is a characteristic of highly integrated and long established families' identity. This could be for reasons of employment, distance, family commitments, at a considerable cost to some individual family members who want to support older relatives with their care needs. Many of these themes are at least partially echoed by Lewis and Glennerster (1996) Means and Smith (1998a) and Chapel (2001) and also in recent policy discourse such as modernisation of social care (DoH 1998a): social inclusion within the community, family capacity building and renewal and social solidity. Family norms and values are potential towards new paradigm and delivery of a new face of the wider welfare system and her is a quote by a family caregiver:

I mean the fact that he's like that, it's very upsetting... it's upsetting for both of us... all the things we were going to do when we retired, and we never could, here we are still together I can't walk away can I? Strangers would not understand what we are going through; therefore, you cannot rely on them... would you.

The care model has the ability to nurture capacity among older relatives, families and communities. This is surely core strength of family reciprocity; recognising the key roles those older relatives and their families have to play in shaping and providing services. This is from the teenager to adult and also the over 65 year siblings, who can all play a major part in care giving and support to relatives in later life (Delaney and Delaney 2003; Lewis 2004; Glendinning 2008, 2009). The future of the care model is about family empowerment, choice and control, individually tailored provision of care to older people in their own home and increased capacity in the wider social care market. However, stress of care giving could be a factor that may endanger the aspirations of families in care giving: adherence to strict values and routines, as well as fear of the unknown can create undue stress when circumstances challenge caregivers to take risks and be adaptable (Lewis and Glennerster 1996; Lister 2001; Carers National Association 2001).

In a similar vein, Wistow et al (2000a) explain the need, demand, expectations, values and governance arrangements, which might be expected to apply, some two decades ahead. This book attempts to project, from current experiences and aspirations, a coherent vision of the purposes and shape of older people services to be achieved.By definition, it seeks to establish a desired destination for older people services as a result of policy and implementation processes which are currently in place such as the modernisation of social services (DoH 1998a; Blair 1998a). The level of public and political debate on social care for older people in our society is on the whole, inadequately informed and often trivial (Wilkinson 1998; Wanless Report 2006; Joseph Rowntree Foundation 2007, 2009).

Too often, older people are discussed in terms of a problem population, presenting a threatening economic burden to current and future generations. They are also often talked about as if they are members of the same homogenous group, bound together; above all, by the number of years they carry (Phillipson et al 2001). Little acknowledgement is made of their considerable diversity, unlike that offered to those within working age or children in our society.Different levels of wealth and poverty, the range of cultural aspiration and practice, variations in health and frailty, will influence the way in which the different needs and wishes of older relatives are manifested (Phillipson et al 1986; Phillipson 1990; Giddens 1998; Glendinning et al 2008).

The ideology of this care model considers the future of older people services by applying family theory on the basis of assumptions rooted in the past and, or the present, which may be more or less comprehensive and more or less explicit. Even if the consequences of the mixed economy of social care now and in future had been correctly predicted, it would still have been necessary to shape and re-shape these forces in accordance with explicit views about what constituted desirable outcomes (Walker 1998; Wistow et al 2000a). The changing demography, political and economic analysis is needed in order to redesign and deliver a person centred approach for older relatives (Royal Commission on Long-Term Care 1999; Commission for Social Care Inspectorate 2006a &c).

Rethinking Social Policy and Services for Older People

Personalisation of services and family directed support care systems is aimed to re-shape, as well as pointing towards the future care for older relatives. It raises the question of choice and what constitutes desirable directions and destination. In other words, it requires at least a minimal framework of principles and purposes to guide not only the consistent development of policy and practice, but also to provide a reference point for scrutiny, review and revision. Means and Smith (1995, 98) and Walker (1984, 98) advanced the principle of empowerment through users' involvement and provide a useful example of why such frameworks and processes are necessary. While user engagement and empowerment have undoubtedly become more fully developed over the last twenty years in social care, there is also much evidence to demonstrate that they are not rooted in everyday routines and practices, moreover as the baby boomers are entering the social care market. Older people are constrained to undertake their holistic functional activities of daily living because of ageing, frailty, and disabilities, thus family's involvements would help to design their individual programme plan capable to meet their care needs (Sale and Leason 2004)

Thus, it could be argued that core values, principles and objectives in services for older people have undoubtedly become more common in present day personal social services and their significance better understood in the process of building the framework. The current shortage of both formal carers and social workers provides an opportunity to learn about the needs of older people and to combine objectives with the capacity to deliver services (Essex Social Services 2007).This is in line with Wanless Report (2006), who argued the need for social services to develop capacity planning as a necessary contribution to build an ordinary life in practice to sustain the increasing needs of older people. It is, however, questionable whether social workers are even now equipped with sufficient background in theory and practice of care management and especially its applications to their own particular contexts and environments.

Before beginning to identify a more specific set of aims and objectives to provide direction for the care pathway, it is important to consider in a little more detail, the principal forces which will shape development of the model, and those that will continue to have significant influences on the aims and objectives of social care for older people. Family's participation in assessment and care giving could also confidently be expected to remain relevant into the foreseeable future. This understanding coincides with Webb and Weston (1982), Wistow (2005) and Phillpson et al (2001) views of family theory and care giving. This meant that involvement of family members in assessment and care to older relatives could be the answer to the shortage of carers and social workers in meeting the increasing demand for care by the growing older people population. Personalisation and family directed support care services would embody a wider conception of social services directed to the wellbeing of the whole family as well as the community and not only the vulnerable in society social casualties. Herewith is a statement by a family caregiver:

> You know I've lived with him for a long time. No one knows him better than I do... I will like to carry out his needs assessment and care for him because he can be an actor sometimes... I know my father well and have been caring for him since he became ill and unable to care for himself. I think I can draw up his needs from memory. His needs change every day therefore assessment I think is ongoing depending on his mood.

Such a conception would be a complementary service to the collective welfare state, in which the family and the wider community will participate frequently. The care model concept is about families' participation in care needs assessment, planning, organisation and providing care for their older relatives for payment. This philosophy goes beyond the type of informal care of individualism and family orientated care, for which Fowler (1984) argued. Thus, this book advocate that family directed support care systems would stimulate the social care market as a result; families could access it freely without much interference by the state. The families would be empowered to take charge of their older relatives' care needs, and this approach would certainly relieve pressure on the state and rejuvenate family reciprocity. This level of argument supported Blair (1998a), Wilkinson (1998) and Levin-Leigh (2002) discussions about family care giving and enabling powers bestowed by Parliament to the local authorities to sustain community care for older people. This development is illuminated on the grounds of the following perspectives: family democracy, identification of needs and above all to reduce the rigidity enshrined in the Fair Access to Care (DoH 2002) such as critical, substantial, moderate and low needs.

Exploration of Personalisation and Family Care Giving

The themes are intended to question the validity and credibility of the contemporary service frameworks and also to make contributions to address some of the set backs within the system. Thus, are social services and the existing service frameworks likely to facilitate the achievement of these outcomes? The answers to these questions will be linked to the concept of reciprocal family care network and swinging market philosophy (see below). If the concept of the family care needs assessment and care giving for payment was considered, this book in its wisdom has highlighted three dimensions that are core to develop a complementary service framework that could work in parallel with the existing models namely: the family, community and governance.Personalisation of services for older relatives and reinvention of family reciprocity is intended to enhance the autonomy of all the family members that wish to be involved in the decision-making relating to care needs assessment and care giving for older relatives. However, reciprocal family care giving and valued lifestyles each have implications for the wider society. According to Wilkinson (1998), autonomy of all stakeholders and the family care giving are both potential challenges to the traditional conception held by both the family and the wider community. Such challenges will be reinforced by continuing trends in social care and demographic change, more especially, geographic mobility of some families (Evandrous et al 2001). However, here is a quote by a family caregiver:

> I think caring for your older relatives is a sort of social responsibility. Well, I don't see any problem for a payment to family members caring for their older parents. Payment in my own opinion will strengthen social responsibility and your commitment to continuing care for your older relatives.

It is therefore possible that the more autonomy and interdependence are realised as outcomes for older relatives, the more they would expose them to risks which their families, social network and the wider community will find difficult to accept (Raynes et al 2001; Lewis 2006). This philosophy is instrumental leading to the reconstruction of an assessment and care model capable to accommodate the interests of all the key stakeholders in 21st century care provision for older people in the community. The

145

assessment and care structure is represented below and the author called it reinvention of family assessment and care:

Personalisation of Services and Reinvention of Family Care Model

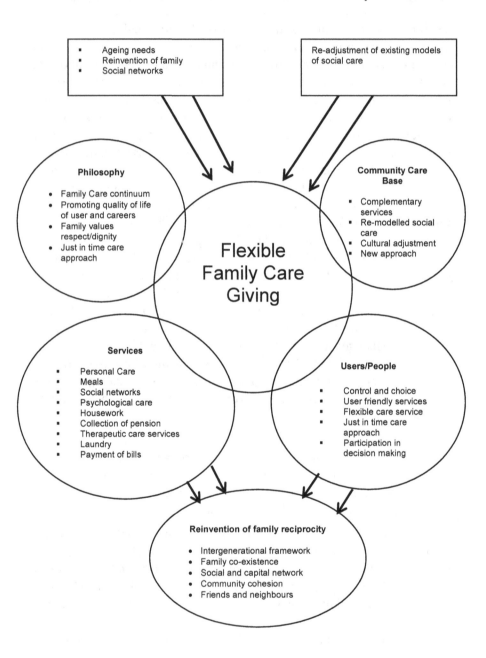

Personalisation of services and reciprocal family care giving is centred on three main psychological understandings namely: Care design in conjunction with the older relative; emotional and psychological support; personal care giving and practical tasks. This multi - dimensional activities differentiated the care model from the existing care pathways of direct managed service, direct payments, and individual budgets. Family care giving would create the atmosphere of social networking, active communications and shared family values and history, which could help to re-establish family reciprocity. This approach is therefore in contrast with the Fair Access to Care (DoH 2002) that demonstrates the levels of care social services can or cannot respond to; critical, substantial, medium, and low. The limit set by most local authorities meant that any referral that is not within critical or substantial matrix will be regarded as an unmet need (Essex Social Services 2002a, b; DoH 2002; Haslar 2006). As a result, attention is not focused on the preventative elements of social care.

Personalisation of services and reciprocal family care giving would be a part of the preventative approach to reduce the increasing social care needs and complaints from service users and their families.The model indicated the strengths and opportunities family direct support would advance in the lives of older relatives both in practical tasks and support systems which sometimes are associated with personal care while practical tasks usually involve contacts that embody the process of care giving. Whenever personal care was provided, it is the only care giving activity that was measured and these echoed previous studies such as Qurush and Walker (1989), Darton et al (2003), Family care needs assessment and care giving for payment might trigger greater public debate to establish what may be termed the social limits to risks in this context. This could raise the issue of boundaries between family relationships and family loyalty pertaining to reciprocity.

Thus, exploration of such issues is an essential element in building a degree of public confidence and community acceptance necessary to underpin reciprocal family care giving. Phillipson et al 2001 argued that the interdependence of older people as a desired and successful outcome has collective implications, in the sense that the ability of individual older relatives to maintain and regain their independence appears to be related to the quality and quantity of their family and social networks as providers of emotional and practical support. In other words, it has implications for social services in terms of understanding, attitudes and behaviours. It would be desirable to review established service frameworks and recognise the need for re-defining the frameworks as domiciliary care through interdependence and social integration with families and the wider community.

More specifically, personalisation of services and family reciprocity would mean: the renewal of the family care giving, an approach that will help to reduce social exclusion and improve family cohesion, family democracy and accountability and renewal of neighbourhood in areas with high levels of deprivation. Reinvention of family reciprocity would strengthen what Alcock (1998) called local governance, which has three benefits such as inclusiveness; as opposed to exclusion, social network and redefinition of older people agenda and these would help older relatives to come to terms with their care needs. It is a contemporary expression of Seebohm's (1968) development agenda for the community as a whole system, where family members would be fully involved in their older relatives care. It also represent community characteristics fundamental to enabling the personal fulfilment of wellbeing of the individual and the groups for whom social care has special responsibilities. This is supported by a comment made by a family caregiver:

> I have lived with my mum throughout my life and I know her, I understand her needs and I cannot go wrong in identifying her needs. I think I am in a position to assess her needs and draw up a flexible programme of care that would meet her needs. I don't think that social workers would understand my mum's needs by just spending one or two hours assessing her needs... that's not realistic.

In reality, these represent a desired outcome of social care for older relatives, both in terms of the general role in the building of community capacity and also the contribution of that capacity to the lifestyles of those who are over 65 years old, with particular needs and requirements. The approach advocates that older relatives, families, social networks and whole community roles are fully interdependent in terms of realising each of the three categories of the outcomes in meeting the needs of older people in their own home (Raynes et al 2001). One of the strengths of the service framework is that it places greater emphasis on developing a holistic perspective on the family care giving in relation to meeting the needs of their older relatives for payment, a move to secure their own economic wellbeing, promoting community involvement and provision of services in older relative's own home (Wistow et al 2002a),.

In line with Jutras and Veilleux (1991) and Allen and Porkins (1995), family care network would facilitate: The whole person perspective, in terms of older people's needs and their wishes, together with the physical, social and psychological factors that shape their abilities for interdependent living in their own home or with their relatives. The family care governance to older relatives in terms of both a comprehensive range of services and an interdependent network of interventions, interact in ways that make such forms of domiciliary living possible. Family directed support care philosophy recognises that individual older people rarely sustain holistic lifestyles in isolation from the social network, which not only promotes physical and mental wellbeing, also and in consequence, makes domiciliary living valued and sustained. In other words family care giving that attracts payment would help to promote, pursue, restore and sustain family relationships (Delaney and Delaney 2003; Wilkinson 1998, 2000). To determine the effectiveness of the family care giving and reciprocity, it is worthwhile examining the argument for social care systems with a view to address the shortage of social care workers.

Conclusion

This chapter centres on the explanatory content of the family care giving; psychological perspective to personalisation and later life care for older people and the exploration of personalisation and reciprocal family care giving for payment. The chapter highlighted a number of advantages, which are not in existence within the contemporary service frameworks such as direct payments, cash for care and direct provision. The joint ownership, family control and choice of care approach have been found to give an important boost to the lives of older people and their families. It may be argued that this framework has some similarities with the current service frameworks, but the difference is that some older people may not be capable as most adult service users with disabilities, to take control and make decisions about their care. Joint decision making with their families is essential. In addition, the chapter identified some challenges within the framework.

Chapter Seven:
Family Care Giving and the Social Care Market

Introduction

A key test for personalisation of services and family care systems for adult and older relatives would be to demonstrate that each of these approaches are realised in practice. It is in this respect that the nature of the relationship between the stakeholders is important. In practice, the tension between the stakeholders is evident, due to shortage of caregivers, social workers and budget constraints. Personal social care and the process of delivery is often an integral part of the outcome. Wistow and Hardy (1998) argued that the way in which services are delivered is an important outcome of social care. Practice observations has indicated that service users place high value on characteristics of care such as kindness, caring attitude of carers, respect for dignity, reliability, unhurried care, consistency and continuity of care and carers. This has lead to the design and construction of what the author called "swinging social care market philosophy".This approach would help to address some of the difficulties and reinforces active family participation in designing personalised services for older relatives:

The swinging market approach will redress the deficits of direct provision, individual budgets and direct payments models of care. The concept seeks to develop a family orientated care continuum, where social services would only intervene as a last resort in those families that are willing to participate in their older relatives care giving. Family care systems would be flexible and performs dual roles to accommodate the interests of the family and social services, which is lacking with the present perspectives.

The criticisms of the existing care models were that families are prevented from assessing and at the same time providing care for their older relatives for payment. Choices of who provides care were limited and that triggered waiting for assessment and care giving to older relatives. The swinging market concept will create elasticity of care giving, which is useful in describing a care-giving pendulum that oscillates between family care giving and managed service. The concept is emerged as part of the contemporary service framework for adult and older people when compared with the traditional social care model. This chapter is narrated within two sub-sections: 1) Personalisation of service and the social care market. 2) Personalisation and the swinging market as applied to family care giving.

Personalisation of Service and the Social Care Market

In support of this argument, personalisation of services and reinvention of family care systems are aimed to promote a swinging market concept i.e. a free market that gives older relatives and their families the flexibility to compare and contrast the social care packages that are available on the market; for example, domiciliary, residential and nursing. The service users and their family would be in a position to make choices of what care packages would meet their holistic care needs. The growing older people's population, now and in future would mean a rethinking of social care pathways currently available to meet the challenges (Royal Commission on Long Term-Care 1999; Commission for Social Care Inspectorate 2006a). This would give rise for the family care giving to be recognised as one of the core approaches to address the shortage of both formal caregivers and social workers in the market. The swinging concept would attempt to recast older people and their families as consumers with choices and this is supported by a statement made by a family caregiver:

> We see mum's care as a family responsibility. My sister as well as her family and my own family joined together to care for mum and that is what she wants and that is how our family history is... This meant that knowing the carer who regularly provides care could be an enduring strength for continuing care.

A reformed social care market could lead to greater emphasis on quality of care giving, person centred approach, education and learning process between the stakeholders. The approach would strengthen the economic concept of: demand and supply, choice and control, service availability, accessibility and accountability in the market. This meant that social services would be in a stronger position to commission care for older relatives through their family caregivers, as well as enabling them to plan and access the social care market of their choice, without interference. This would synchronise with the aspirations of the growing population of older people, who wish their care to be provided in their own home and in the community they know (Raynes et al 2001; Joseph Rowntree Foundation 2009).

Dimensions of the Social Care Market

The NHS and Community Care Act (1990) delegated a duty to social service to meet the assessed care needs within resources availability (s47). Given the circumstances of increasing demand for social care, longevity of older people, the state is the core commissioner of social care for older people. As a result, there is a need for social services, independent sector and families to form a strategic alliance to support personalisation of services and family reciprocity in order to relieve pressure on social services (Blair 1998a; Giddens 1998, Powell 2002). Thus, swinging social care philosophy would facilitate reinvention of family care giving; although the laws of supply and demand would undoubtedly influence the social care market. This meant that no social care model is exempted from market forces of demand and supply, given the limited resources and demographic change in our society (World Bank 2002; UN 1999).

To reduce these uncertainties, the care model would form part of the future social care delivery to address the increasing demand for care from older people. This would enhance capacity and aggregate planning and forecasting future care needs and resource availability in order to tackle the increasing care needs of the growing older people population (Evandrous 1998; Evandrous et al 2001). Family involvement in assessment and care meant that older relatives would not be waiting and there care needs would be met by people they know rather than strangers. Within this level of discussion, financial remuneration to family caregivers is something that would not only bridge the gap and attract, but also renew, the views of the family caregivers in the 21st century and beyond (Glendinning et al 2008, 2009, Wilkinson 2000). This advances the argument in favour of a social care market that promotes flexibility, choice and control beyond which the current service frameworks are dependent on. This would then form part of the political and economic debate of the new phase of the welfare system of the future.

The anticipatory vision of personalisation of services and reinvention of family reciprocity beyond informal care giving meant recognition of economic wellbeing of the family caregivers which in turn would revive family involvement in care giving to older relatives. Given the present economic situation, any family policy that neglects the economic wellbeing of the caregivers would strangulate the enthusiasms of many family caregivers to commit their time and skills for their older relative's care and the flourishment of the market (Hughes et al 1999; Qureshi and Walker 1998; Wilkinson 2000; Powell and Hewitt 1998).The present focus on limited service frameworks are endangering the potential and the future of the social welfare market to meet the increasing demand for care by older people (Royal Commission on Long - Term 1999; Commission for Social Care Inspectorate 2006). From practice point of view, despite the recommendations of the NHS and Community Care Act (1990), social services are failing to fully engage the family caregivers and social capital such as friends, neighbours and voluntary sector organisations as partners in responding to shortages of both social workers and formal carers.In view of the inflexibility in the social care market, swinging social care model would rejuvenate the market:

Swinging Social Care Market as Applied to Family Care Giving

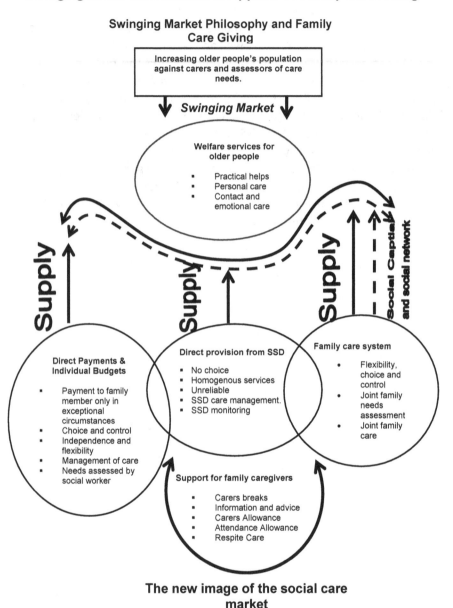

Swinging Market Philosophy and Family Care Giving

Increasing older people's population against carers and assessors of care needs.

Swinging Market

Welfare services for older people

- Practical helps
- Personal care
- Contact and emotional care

Supply

Supply

Supply

Social Capital and social network

Direct Payments & Individual Budgets

- Payment to family member only in exceptional circumstances
- Choice and control
- Independence and flexibility
- Management of care
- Needs assessed by social worker

Direct provision from SSD

- No choice
- Homogenous services
- Unreliable
- SSD care management.
- SSD monitoring

Family care system

- Flexibility, choice and control
- Joint family needs assessment
- Joint family care

Support for family caregivers

- Carers breaks
- Information and advice
- Carers Allowance
- Attendance Allowance
- Respite Care

The new image of the social care market

The swinging market concept is about redoubling of efforts by the social services to strengthen the mixed economy of social care, including among other things: educating the families about modernisation of social services and redesigning of personal services for older relatives, family reciprocity and traditional family care, providing the family with accurate information about resource availability, financial support to family caregivers and effective campaign and recruitment of family caregivers (Modernising Social Services (DoH) 1998a; Royal Commission on Long-Term Care 1999; Pearson 2006; Haslar 2006; Glendinning et al 2009).

> My mother is the main carer for my father. But my sister and I negotiate how best to support my father and my mother in her caring role. We all sit down together, plan and think things through, the best care for my father. We grieve together, we socialise together because we are a family.

The concept of swinging market would provide a buffer to both social service and users/families in times of increased pressure and stress to continue care giving. It is termed a swinging market because the users and their families have at least various options and choices available any giving time and could switch services within the market as family circumstances changed. The model and structure is developed to demonstrate the operations and functions of the future image of the social market and swinging market approach would feature prominently. The diagram below represents a comparison between the service frameworks:

The opportunity to access the social care market would give families and users the choice to evaluate the type and qualities of social care products (Domiciliary care, day care, residential or nursing care placements) available to be tapped into in times of potential pressures and crisis in the family. The market would also offer the family caregivers the opportunity to have a break and rebuild their efforts to continue care giving for their older relatives. The interactions in the market have the propensity to promote continuity of care giving, carers breaks and quality assurance during care giving and reduce the risk of care breakdown.

The service framework provides the recipe for social services to concentrate in policy formulations, planning, developing and commissioning packages of care that are appropriate to meet the aspirations of older people in the 21st century and beyond. Thus, allowing the current service frameworks run their course in the wider welfare systems meant a significant under utilisation of family untapped human resources. These views echo Blair (1997a, 98a), Carers National Association (2001), and Help the Aged (2002) who in their respective roles and campaign advocate for family involvement in their older relative care management. The inclusion of families and social network would in part see a new dimension that could facilitate swinging care market within the wider welfare system.

Thus, this care model should be seen as an innovative systems approach and one councillor stated:

> This provides the opportunity to embrace the Big Society agenda and personalisation of services for older people in their own home directed by their family members. That's what I call innovation... I think. Therefore any extra income to the family would act as an inducement to many... those within lower socio-economic classes.

Modernisation of services for older people and the swinging market approaches would present some challenges to the monopolistic or imperfect markets that exist at present in the welfare service, a system where choices are restricted to few service frameworks (Help the Aged 2002; Glendinning et al 2009). The perspective is also in contrast with a quasi market; a market where social services negotiates and buys health and social care on behalf of the users, although the market functions in two tiers. Social services on the one hand represent the interest of those services users that do not have enough money, to buy care privately for themselves. On the other hand, service users who have enough money can approach service providers directly and pay for their care (Wanless Report 2006).

With the swinging market perspective, families would come to an agreement with social services to switch care giving when they are unable to continue care giving for their older relatives, because of family circumstances. Personalisation of care for older relatives would in part help them achieve their wish to be cared for by the people they know and who are committed to assist them with their care needs in their own home (Lewis 2004; Glendinning et al 2008). According to Commission for Social Care Inspectorate (2006a) and Carers National Association (2001), family care giving could be cost effective for social services, because payment to family caregivers above the minimum wage would still be less than the declared rates paid to independent provider agencies. Moroney (1976) argued that the danger of failing to reconsider economic inducement to family caregivers will endanger the personal social services and he notes:

> By not offering support to family caregivers, existing social policy might actually force many families to give up this function prematurely, given the evidence of the severe strain many families, social workers and the social services are experiencing. If this were to happen, the family and the state would not be sharing the responsibilities through an interdependent

relationship and it's conceivable that eventually the welfare system would be pressurised with demands to provide even greater amounts of care, to become the family for more and older people (Moroney 1976).

Certainly, at one level, personalisation of services, directed by family members would reflect commitment and collaboration between social services and family caregivers. Social care for older relatives would constantly change as ideas emerged and developed about the strengths and weaknesses of different service frameworks through which publicly funded social care delivered. Such options would expand as older people are living longer, becoming highly dependent and exercising their human rights as other citizens of the state (Evandrous et al 2001; United Nations 2002). For older people to utilise fully the contemporary service frameworks of individual budgets or direct payments schemes, family members would have to be a core stakeholder to make it work. This is because people are living longer and as a result some does not have the capabilities or strength to take on the responsibilities needed to organise their own care needs. In most cases, it is left for the family members to advocate and participate in their older relatives holistic care needs delivery (Pearson 2006; Haslar 2006; Hunter and Ritchie 2007).

In whatever way social care is provided, it will reflect political, economic and social values. Community care reforms are based upon a desire to minimise the service delivery role of social services directed towards a radical decentralisation of decision-making and service delivery within social services (Walker 1995; Organisation for Economic Co-operations and Developments 1998). Social care reforms needs to reflect the changing demography, the increasing older people's population, social networks and social capital within society. Demographic mobility in some families, smaller family units, changing economic situations in some families and pursuit of employment is likely to influence the families' ability and opportunities to provide care for their older relatives (Office for National Statistics 2001; World Bank 2002; O'Hara 2004).

Personalisation of services for older relatives and reinvention of family reciprocity beyond informal care relationships would promote closer caring relationships between the cared for person, the family and social service, which would in turn reduce waiting for care and complaints for poor quality of care. The approach stands to create awareness, promoting and campaigning for family involvement in order to promote more choices in the social care market. Family's participation in assessment and care would contribute to partnership and joint working between the stakeholders thus, resulting in lateral thinking, advice and information, crisis intervention, and carers' short term breaks (Clarke and Glendinning 2002; UN 2002; Lewis 2003, 05). According to Duncan-Smith (2010), the growth of older people in our society poses a threat to both the national and local government; therefore, an urgent measure is needed to address their increasing demand for services.

Policy shift towards family care giving would synchronise with recent research findings (Carvel 2006, 2007) which indicated that the users of home care; be it private, independent and public provision nationally is forecasted to grow by up to 65% between 2001 to 2031 and this will place more pressure on social services to meet their care needs. During the same period; Carvel (2007) states that informal caregivers would progressively decline by 0.5% annually, due to economic migration, women in search of full time employment and ageing spouses. The gap in the social care market will strengthen the debate for personalisation of services and family reciprocity, although this may have moral and cultural implications to some users and the caregivers (Qureshi et al 2002).

Reciprocal family care giving appears to be a viable preposition for now and in the future to tackle the growing older people's population, since the baby boomers are becoming older and may be needing care services in their own right, therefore would be unable to support older relatives (Evandrous et al 2001; Carvel 2007). The UN concludes:

> We live in a changing world where sociology, science and technology are embedded into our daily functional activities. This leaves national governments to be proactive in order to accommodate and meeting its delegated duties and powers within the welfare service (the UN 2002a).

Insights and Modernisation of Social Care

Modernisation of public services and the wider welfare systems have paved the way to review conventional service frameworks, policy and practice dimensions relevant to long-term care for the growing older people. In addition, demographic change, constriction of formal care systems and longevity of care giving to older people has triggered the need for a debate towards a new paradigm. Thus, the stance of this book is to argue in support for re-evaluation of the present care pathways of direct provision, direct payments and individual budgets through: 1) Re-arrangement of patterns of care for older people. 2) Paradigm shift within social policy for older people and the role of the professionals and family members. 3) Identifying the skills and knowledge to achieve community care for older people. 4) Bridging the gap between assessment and care within the welfare system. These bring us back to questions concerning the effectiveness of social policy for adult and older people's services and the commissioning of social care now and the future. Thus, this chapter is concluded within the following themes: personal social services and welfare perspectives; personalisation and knowing the person providing care and policy and practice dimensions.

Personal Social Services and Welfare Perspectives

Linking with the conventional care systems, the questions are "does the apparent persistence of both problems and solutions in services for older people suggest that the implementation of the Seebohm Report (Donnison 1968) and the National Health Service and Community Care Act (DoH 1990) were a failure, or rather that it failed to be implemented?"Thus, the question reinforces the fact that any discussions of the aims and objectives of the service frameworks should take into account the imperfect relationship between demand and supply within the social care market on the one hand, and implementation of policies such as the Community Care Act and modernisation of services for older people now and in the future (Glennerster 2006). To further the discussion, it is appropriate to return to the concept of choice and developing a provider mix. These concepts formed the basis of the National Health Service and Community Care legislation (DoH 1990) and managed markets (Quasi Market) within a mixed economy of care (Griffiths 1988; Walker 1982 & 1995; DoH 1998a). Linking this with social work practice the stakeholders (older people, family caregivers and social workers) re-affirmed that there were fundamental difficulties about the operation of the social care market. Unlike the purchaser choice for most consumer goods, a shift to family care giving for payment (beyond the carers allowance) is not yet an option.

Social services have little previous knowledge to guide or inform these choices and the practice observations conclude the inadequacies within the social care market. Choices are control because of inconsistent costs regulations and the imbalance between demand and supply in the market. The market is still developing and the slow pace of developments is restricting choice and control leading to inequitable service provisions. The king's Fund (2005) advocates for a working and practical social care market and their views were based on the concept of choice in social care, which is problematic for at least two reasons: 1) The conditions, which give rise to individuals and families needing to access services, may mitigate against the exercise of choice and control in the social care market. 2) The decisions about access to social care are in most cases relatively rare lifetime events, but the growth of older people population and their longevity would potentially increase the likelihood of needing social care in the future. Individual decision making over direct provision, direct payments, cash for care or individual budgets added to delays in care provision because of the uneven distribution of social care providers, all of whom have waiting allocations

Previous studies and reports demonstrated the issues concerning professional dominance in decision making regarding choices for domiciliary care giving in the community. In the present social work practice (Lymbery 2004; Pearson 2006), most service users argued that social workers were unable to give older people a choice of social care package because availability was a problem, both in-house and in the independent sector. The domiciliary care services were characterised by a high eligibility criteria (Fair Access to Care - DoH 2002), limited access at key times of the day and a considerable shortage of supply in the independent sector for more routine support services such as day and respite care, as well as sitting service.

Family directed support care systems would promote a strategic alliance with social services in order to address the un-met needs within the older people's service. On reflection, Leadbeater (2004) and Hunter and Ritchie (2007) argued that increasing demand for care from service users has created the need for personalisation and co-production of care for users. It is hoped that this approach would promote choice and control in the social care market. Older people and their family would be in a better position to choose who, where and how their care would be provided and they would participate in the design of their care and be in control for as long as they are able to do so. The user and their family would be central in the delivery of care in the community. Social services are faced with the question of how best to safeguard the human and material resources provided by the family.

Resources have not been carefully monitored despite the assertion to the contrary in some legislation (such as the NHS and Community Care Act (DoH 1990), the National Service Framework for Older People (DoH 2001a) and the Commission for Social Care Inspectorate (2006a). Thus, the family directed support care system would facilitate long-term planning, organising and providing care for their older relatives for payment within the wider community and society in general. Care giving to older relatives and the challenges this presents is now beyond what one agency can adequately meet. This has some correlation with modernisation agenda of pluralistic vision of care delivery such as highlighted in the, private finance initiatives

(PFI), partnership, collaboration and joint working initiatives between the stakeholders in the wider welfare system (Blair 1998a; Callaghan 2003). While the modernisation - partnership and personalisation of services lead by family members is intended to enhance shared responsibilities and family/service users' empowerment and participation. There would be an increasing awareness of policy differences and performance indicators between agencies (Lister 2001; Pearson 2006).

However, there are potential tendencies, which could mean that some agencies within the partnership would be overshadowed and relegated to passive partners. The problem identified by Lister (2001) as well as the King's Fund (2006) and the Commission for Social Care Inspectorate (2006a) is that service provider organisations are not necessarily free from exploitations, either by implication or negligence. Therefore greater understanding is needed to ensure all stakeholders are well informed and represented in decision making regarding criteria for needs assessment, budget allocations, implementation of policies and controlling of resources.

Familiarity of care needs and Providing Care

Knowing the person providing care would promote personalisation of care through co-designing and provision of care between the older relative and the family. This would enable the older relatives to see themselves as individuals who have rights, choices and opportunities to achieve their aspirations in life. Practice observation has shown that most service users and family caregivers acknowledged the limitations of strangers having to provide care to older relative. Strangers have limited time available and they are unable to offer quality care to service users, and this could be depressing and frustrating (Hunter and Ritchie's 2007). Family caregivers know the standards of care their older relatives are used to and would endeavour to facilitate that.This means that family care giving would promote person centred care, giving the users the opportunity to enjoy their holistic functional activities of daily living, like any other person. Family members could present a forum for personalisation of services and co-production of social care capable of meeting functional activities of daily living of their older relative in their own home. Familiarity of needs and providing care would create the opportunity for rapport, compliance and participation and these would reduce the risk of care breakdown, as all concerned are active partners. A social worker summarised the perspective as follows:

> The family will have a plan and build the care plan within their overall daily activities and they will make sure, that their

relative will not be left unsupported as and when required. You will always recognise your family and you will always rely on them for your needs, this cannot be the same with strangers... Continuity to me is about having care continuum.

Reconstituted policy framework in favour of the traditional family directed social care for older relative would help reduce waiting times for assessment and care, acute hospital bed blocking and antagonistic relationships between social workers and family members. It could equally reduce re-imbursement charges (DoH 2003; Lymbery 2004) and enable social workers to concentrate on core and complex care management. The family caregivers would be involved from the beginning, planning and providing care for their older relatives as soon as possible. Such an early intervention would reduce stress, anxiety, frustration and would promote psychosocial wellbeing amongst the users and their family members. The older relatives would be assured that they would not be seeing different faces visiting them to offer care, and they would not be repeating themselves all the time to explain their care plan to strangers.

This opportunity would enhance family relationships, as they would be in a better position to share their family norms and values, history and culture (Gallagh-Thmpson and Powers 1997). Previous studies such as Lewis and Glennerster (1996) and Wilkinsion (1999, 2000) stressed the importance of family involvement in care giving and community wellbeing for older people. Practice experience has shown that family members would offer person centred care approach in addition, through talking and listening attentively to the holistic care needs of their older relatives far beyond what formal caregivers or professionals could offer. Talking to the cared for person during care giving can be therapeutic and might contribute to quick recovery, re-orientation to the environment, time for building a good rapport between the cared for person and the caregiver. The families would play a crucial role in the system by assuming responsibilities and being accountable for their part in the process and this would reduce blame culture.Below is a comment from a service user:

Familiarity of needs and providing care would improve response time for care as well as assistance or support to cope with difficult situations during care giving. It would also reduce anxiousness, communication breakdown and complaints from the families.

Policy and Practice Dimensions

Family-directed support and care giving could reshape the view held by many people that only the state should be responsible for meeting the holistic needs of older people (Carvel 2006 & 2007). Opinion poll (Carvel 2007) has shown that family care giving would strengthen policy and practice in delivering care to older people in their own homes. This echoed some of the Commission for Social Care Inspectorate's (2006a) view that direct provision and direct payments are increasingly challenged by recent developments in the social care market, in particular by the apparent increase in demand for home care from older people and their families. Families' engagement in care giving to older relatives would determine the pace at which social services could meet the increasing demand for care.

This approach could influence policy and political dimensions with implementation being for the benefit of all stakeholders. Policy and political philosophy in relation to community care has developed largely by default (Townsend 1983; Walker 1995; Glennerster 1983 & 2006). While the perverse incentive created by social security policies in the past has been debated, politicians have been unwilling to engage in a more wide ranging debate on complementary domiciliary care (The Royal Commission on Long-Term Care for Older People 1999; Wanless Report 2006). This pointed out the gross negligence of other policy issues such as the relative responsibilities of local authorities to engage families as complementary to a state-dominant approach. The above argument could be supported by a quote from a family caregiver:

> Current changes in social services are long overdue in my opinion... family care giving... is a new idea within the industry as I see it... It could bring about things like choice, control and a focus within the wider community care. Family care giving I hope would change the way we do things now and projects future social work and social care for service users.

A significant number of research such as Lewis (2004), Twigg and Atkin (1994) and Glendinning et al (2009) thought the caring role of families should be acknowledged and supported, given the increase in the size of the older people population and of the staff shortages in the social care market. The stakeholders, especially the family caregivers, advocated a paradigm shift involving giving families more responsibilities to decide about and participate in their older relatives' care. The perspective would change the policy and practice held dearly by social services and social workers that only the state can deliver quality care to the vulnerable in society. The growing older people population over the of 75 years old indicates a burden on society (Evandrous et al 2001; O'Hara 2004), a group with the potential for reducing the living standards of the nation and increasing the financial pressures on future generations of workers. In 1999, a second Royal Commission on Long-Tern Care for Older People repeated the dilemmas that the growing number of older people would pose to the state if no action were taken to address the issues.

Thus, family directed support care systems signals a complementary service that would be useful to have developed in support of current service frameworks. The approach would not only enrich the conventional care models but would be a menu for behavioural and policy change at both micro and macro policy levels in social services over the long-term care for older people.The care model would be an added opportunity for social services to tap into in order to reduce over reliance on direct managed services (Wilkinson 1999, 2000; Finch 1995). Traditional family care system is a vehicle towards shared responsibilities and resource re-distribution amongst all stakeholders. This is supported by a quote from a family caregiver:

> A family member is with that person and sees it from a much more personal level... you know sometimes family members have more of an overview of the quality of life the person has been maintaining. Strangers however may have a different idea of what is required... what his/her life should be or can be... so that would be good.

The increasing demand for care from older people and their support systems requires a more committed strategy and policy where families would be more involved and take a lead role (Wilkinson 1998, 99, 2000). Thus, collaborative working between the family and the state should work in parallel, ensuring that holistic functional activities of older people were met by mobilising the wisdom of all the key stakeholders in full. Well-informed families might not wish to approach social services for care and support, since they would know what they wanted. Most families would like to persevere and source their needs amongst themselves and be independent of social services for as long as possible (Wilkinson 2000).

However, demographic and socio-economic change has made the achievement of this aim socially more difficult today; as a result a combined effort between the key stakeholders might make it possible to develop a capable workforce to arrest the development of the impending problems (Evandrous 1998 and Evandrous et al 2001). A new approach has to be found. The care model would facilitate good practice and policy implementations to resolve some of the concerns that were raised by some stakeholders. This would take the form of setting up achievable goals such as proportional assessment of care needs, unequivocal carer's assessment and short term breaks and standards of care provision. These would minimise potential concerns such as abusive situations, burdens on family caregivers and longevity of care giving to older relatives. It would also help to look at how the service overcomes the obstacles to modernisation of social care such as personalisation of services and to find innovative approaches to assessment and care. Good practice and policy framework would facilitate a great opportunity for planning and to get the right care support in place, which would alleviate care breakdowns, poor working relationships between the family caregivers and social workers. The vision would connect decision making between the key stakeholders and focus attention on areas of importance while addressing specific issues and priorities of care delivery.

Enhanced policy and practice would strengthen the commitment for the initial four to six weeks and subsequent annual reviews of care packages. This would potentially help to identify issues of concern earlier and deal with it before it is escalated to major problems such as abuse (physically, finance, deprivation) "No Secret Act" (DoH 2000). Continuous reviews advances the opportunity to re-examine the adequacy of care packages, which might lead to either a decrease or increase in support for the cared for person. Additionally, it paves the way for holistic support to both the user and their family caregiver as and when necessary. These possibilities could reduce the increased burdens, stress, antagonistic relationships between the key stakeholders and the reliance on family caregivers during continuing care to older relatives. Similarly, adherence to policy and legislative frameworks such as Fair Access to Care (DoH 2002) would help to lessen dependency culture because, assessment and care would be commissioned in line with practice and policy guidance and this could reduce complaints.

Concluding summary

One of the aims of personalisation of services for older people and reinvention of family reciprocity is to explore the differences and similarities of the existing service frameworks. The outcome of which would pave the way to map out core services that are capable enough to address the increasing older peoples increasing demand for care. The anticipatory assumption for reciprocal family care giving has highlighted a number of advantages, which are not in existence within the contemporary service frameworks. The joint ownership, family control and choice of care approach have been found to give an important boost to the lives of older people and their families. In the event, family's intervention to undertake care needs assessment and care provision for payment would advance community care for older people to a different level forestall by the ethos ofthe community care legislation. To offer older people the best possible social care, it could be argued that joint decision making with their families is essential. In addition to the potential of the family care giving, this book has identified some challenges within the framework.

This book embraces policy and practice dimensions such as personalisation of services for adult and older relatives and marketisation of services within the welfare systems. The care model could also be one of the ways in which to deliver the modernisation and embrace the "Big Society" agenda within the adult and older people's services. Therefore, a key test for the model would be to demonstrate that policy decisions are achievable in practice. It is in this respect that the nature of the relationship between social services, families/users and the wider community is so important. Personal social services and the process of delivery are often an integral part of the outcome and cannot be separated. The book argued that users of domiciliary care services placed high value on characteristics of care delivery such as reliability, unhurried care, consistency and continuity of care and carers.

References

Allen, I and Perkins, R (1995) The Future of Family Care for Older People. London: HMSO.

Alock, P (1998): Consolidation or Stagnation Social Policy under the Major Government in M. May, E. Brunsden and G. Craig (eds), Social Policy Review of London's Social Policy Association.

Barusch, A. S. (1995). "Programming for Family Care of Elderly Dependents: Mandates, Incentives, and Service Rationing." Social Work 40(3):315–322.

Bauld, L, Chesterman, J, Davies, B, Judge, K and Mangalore, R (2000). Caring for Older people: An Assessment of Community Care in the 1990s, Aldershot, Ashgate.

Bauman, Z. (1990): Thinking Sociologically. Oxford: Blackwell.

Beach, S. R.; Schulz, R.; Yee, J. L.; and Jackson, S. (2000). "Negative and Positive Health Effects of Caring for a Disabled Spouse: Longitudinal Findings from The Caregiver Health Effects Study." Psychology and Aging 15(2):259–271.

Bennett, G and Kingston, P. (1993) Elder Abuse: concepts, theories and interventions. London, Chapman & Hall.

Blair, T (1998a): The Third Way. London. Fabian Society.

Blair, T (1997a): New Labour Because Britain Deserves Better, General Election Manifesto, London: Labour Party.

Breda, J, Shoenmaekers, D, Van Landeghem, C, Claessens, D and Geerts, J (2006) When Informal Care Becomes a Paid Job: the case of Personal Assistantce Budgets in Flanders, in C Glendinning and P. A Kemp (eds), Cash and care: Policy challenges in the welfare state, Policy Press, Bristol, pp 155-170.

Bulger, M. W.; Wandersman, A.; and Goldman, C. R. (1993). "Burdens and Gratifications of Care giving: Appraisal of Parental Care of Adults with Schizophrenia." American Journal of Orthopsychiatry 63(2):255–265.

Burgess, E .E (edn) (1960): Ageing in the Western societies. University of Chicago Press Chicago.

Cameron, D (2010) The Big Society Agenda: The Conservative Party Manifesto 2010.

Callaghan, D (2003) "When two become one" Community Care, 25 September-1st October, pp 34-5.

Campbell, T (1996): Implementing Direct Payments: Towards the next Millennium, National Institute of Social Work Conference, 12 November (1996).

Care Services Improvement Partnership (Department of Health 2006) Commissioning e-book at http://www.cat.csip.org.uk

Carers National Association (1996): Who Cares? Perceptions of Caring and Carers, London: Carers National Association.

Carers National Association (2001): Informal Care. Perceptions of Caring and Carers, London: Carers National Association.

Carey, M. A (2003) Anatomy of a Care Manager, Work Employment and Society, 17, 1 pp 121-35.

Carvel, J (2006): Public Say; Prevention most Important for Ageing Research

A Public Consultation by Ipsos MORI for Research Councils UK.

Public Say

Carvel, J (2007): Prospect of Means to a Care Home Frightens two Thirds of Britons: Growing Old; MOP Guardian Newspapers; March 2007.

Challis D, Hughes J (2002). 'Frail old people at the margins of care: some recent research findings'. British Journal of Psychiatry, vol 180, pp 126–30.

Clarke, J and Glendinning, C (2002) Partnership and the remaking of Welfare Provision, in C Glendinning, M, Powell and K, Rummery (eds) Partnerships, New Labour and the Governance of welfare, Bristol, Policy Press.

Clarke, J Gewertz, S and McLaughlin, E (2000). New Managerialism, New Welfare, London Sage.

Clarke, J, Cochrane, A and McLaughlin (1994): Introduction to Social Policy in J.

Clarke, J, Cochrane A, Smart, C (1987): Ideologies of Welfare, London Hutchinson.

Commission for Social Care Inspection (2005a): The State of Social Care in England 2004-05. London: Commission for Social Care Inspection.

Commission for Social Care Inspection (2005b): Social Services Performance Assessment Framework Indicators 2005-06. London. : Commission for Social Care Inspectorate.

Commission for Social Care Inspection (2006a): Handled with Care? A special Study Report. London. Commission for Social Care Inspection.

Commission for Social Care Inspection (2006b): Professional Advice: The administration of medicines in domiciliary care. London: Commission for Social care Inspection.

Commission for Social care Inspection (2006c): Relentless Optimism. Creative Commissioning for Personalised Care (2006): Report of a Seminar Held by Commission for Social care Inspection on 18th May 2006.

Commission for Social Care Inspection (2006): Delivery and Improvement Statements; Spring (2006) Commission on Social Justice (1994): Social Justice: Strategies for National Renewal, London Vintage.

Coolen, J and Weekers, S (1998): Long Term Care in the Netherlands, Public Funding and Private Provision within a Universalistic Welfare State, in C, Glendinning (eds) Rights and Realities Comparing new Development to Long Term Care for Older People, Bristol: The Policy Press.

Cooney, R S & Di, J (1999): Primary Family Caregivers of Impaired Elderly in Shanghai, China, Research on Ageing 21, 739-761.

Darton R., Netten A., Forder J. (2003):'The cost Implications of the Changing population and Characteristics of Care Homes'. International Journal of Geriatric Psychiatry 18, 236-243.

Delany, S and Delany A. E (2003). Having Our Say: The Delany Sister's First 100 Years. New York: Dell.

Department of Health (1990): National Health Service and Community Care in the next Decade and Beyond: Police Guidance, London DOH.

Department of Health (1996a): Community Care (Direct Payments) Act 1996, Policy and Practice Guidance, London (DOH.)

Department of Health (1996b.): Direct Payment Act: Presentation Materials, London DOH.

Department of Health (1998a): Modernising Social Services CM 4169, London: The Stationery Office.

Department of Health (2000): The NHS Plan: A Plan for Investment, A Plan for Reform, London: HMSO.

Department of Health (2000a): Community Care (Direct Payments) Act 1996: Policy and Practice Guidance (2nd. edn). London, DH.

Department of Health (2000) No Secrets: Guidance on Development and Implementing Multi-Agency Policies and Procedures to Protect Vulnerable Adults from Abuse. Stationary Office. London.

Department of Health (DoH) (2001a) The National Service Framework for Older People, London HMSO.

Department of Health (2001b) Carers and Disabled Children Act (2000) Carers and People with Parental Responsibility for Disabled Children: Policy Guidance, London. Department of Health.

Department of Health (2001d) The Single Assessment Process Consultation Papers and Process, Stationary Office, London.

Department of Health (2002a): Domiciliary Care National Minimum Standards Regulations, London: Department of Health.

Department of Health (2002b): LAC (2002): 13 Fair Access to Care Services. Guidance on Eligibility Criteria for Adult Social Care, London: Department of Health.

Department of Health (DoH) (2003a) The Community Care (Delayed Discharges) Act (2003): Guidance for Implementing, HSC2003/009: LAC (2003) 21, London Department of Health.

Department of Health (2005a): Best Practice Guidance on the Role of the Director of Adult Social Services. London: Department of Health. Department of Health (2005b): Independence, Wellbeing and Choice: Our Vision for the Future of Social Care in England. London: Department of Health.

Department of Health (2006): Our Health, Our Care, Our Say. London: Department of Health.Department for Work and Pensions, Social Exclusion Unit (2006): A Sure Start to Later Life: Ending Inequalities for Older People. Wellbeing Office of the Deputy Prime minister: Publications.

Department of Work and Pensions (2005): Opportunity Age: Meeting the Challenges of Aging in the 21st century'. London: Department of Works and Pensions.

Department of Health (2000): Carers and Disabled Children: Support for Carers. London, HMSO

Department of Work and Pensions (2005): 'Opportunity Age: Meeting the Challenges. London Her Majesty Stationary Office.

Donnison, D (1968): Seebohm.Report and its Implication Social Work 25.4

Dowling. C (1996) Red Hot Mamas: Coming into Our Own at Fifty. New York Bantam.

Essex Social Services (2002): Best Value Review: Older people. Essex County Council.

Essex social Services Review (2002): Social Services Inspectorate. Essex. County Council.

Essex Social Care Report (2007): Working Together for Wellbeing: Delivering the Vision for Adult Social Care: Local Government Association.

European Network on Independent Living (1997): Training on Direct Payments for Personal Assistance, Report from the ENIL Seminar, Berlin, and 1-4 May 2001.

Evandrou, M (Eds) (1998): Baby Boomers: What Future When We Retire? London. Age Concern.

Evandrou, M, Falkingham, J (1998) 'The Personal Social Services'. The state welfare: the Economics of Social Spending, Oxford: Oxford University

Evandrou, M, Falkingham, J, Rake, K and Scott, A. (2001): The Dynamics of Living Arrangements in Later Life: Evidence from the British Household Panel Survey, Population Trends 105:37-44.

Fielding, N (1994): Varieties of Research Interviews. Nurse Researcher 1 (3) p4-13.

Finch, J (1989) Family Obligations and Social Change. Cambridge: Polity.

Finch, J (1995) Responsibilities, Obligations and Commitments, in Allen, I and Perkins, E (eds) The Future of Family Care for Older people. HMSO.

Finch, J and Masson, J (1993) Negotiating Family Responsibilities. London: Routledge.

Gallagher-Thompson, D & Powers, D V (1997): Primary Stressors and Depressive Symptoms in Caregivers of Dementia Patients, Ageing and Mental. Health 1, 248- 255 Ethics in Health and Illness (Ed. P. Benner), pp 43-63 Thousand Oaks. Sage.

Giddens, A (1998) The third Way: The Renewal of Social Democracy. Cambridge. Polity.

Glasby, J and Glasby, J (1999): Paying for Social Services: Social Services and Local Government Finance. Birmingham: Paper Publications.

Glasby, J and Littlechild. R. (2000a): Fighting Times? Emergency Hospital Admission and the Concept of Prevention: Journal of Management in Medicine Volume 14, no 2 pp 109-18.

Glasby, J and Littlechild, R (2000b): The Health and Social Care Fund. The Experiences of Old People Birmingham: Paper Publications.

Glendinning, C, Tjadeens, F, Arksey, H, Moree, M, Moran, N, and Nies, N (2009) Care Provision within Families and its Socio-economic Impact on Care Provisions, Report for the European Commission DG EMPL.

Glendinning, C and Rummery, K (2008) Individualised Budget: Carers Individualised Budget Pilot: Health and Social Care. Bristol Policy Press.

Glendinning, C, Powell, M and Rummery, K eds (2002). Partnerships "New Labour and the Governance of Welfare, Bristol, Policy Press.

Glendinning, C, Haliwell, S, Jacob, S, Rummary, K and Tyne, J (2000a): Buying Independence: Using Direct Payments to Integrate Health and Social Services, Bristol: The Policy Press.

Glendinning, C, Haliwell, S, Jacobs, S, Rummary, K and Tyne, J (2000b): Bridging the Gap: Using Direct Payments to Purchase Integrated Care. Health and Social Care in the Community, Volume 8 no 3 pp 192-200.

Glennerster, H (eds) (2006): British Social Policy; 1945 to the present. Blaclwell Publishing.

Glennerster, H (eds) (1983): The Future of Welfare State, London Heinemann

Gordon, C (1988) The Myth of Family Care? The Elderly in the Early 1930s. London: The Welfare State Programme, London School of Economics.

Griffiths, R (1988): Community Care: An Agenda for Action. London. Her Majesty Stationary Office.

Grundy, E (1991): The Demographic Context of Ageing. The House Magazine 16 (24 June) 19.

Halloran, J (edn) (1998): Towards a People's Europe: A Report on the Development of Direct Payments in 10 Member States of the European Union. Vienna: European Social Network.

Hasler, F (2006). The Direct Payments Development Fund, in Leece, J and Bornat, J (eds) (2006) Development in Direct Payments, Bristol Policy Press

Hasler, F (2000): What is Direct Payments in J Britt, T Bignall and E Stone (Eds), Directing Support: Report from a Workshop on Direct Payments and Black and Minority Ethnic Eligible People York, Joseph Rowntree. Foundation

Hasler, F, and Zarb. G (2000): Direct Payments and Older People: Social Services. University of York Press.

Hayman, H (1954): Interviewing in Social Research. Chicago: University press.

Health and Social Care (Community Health and Standards) Act 2003 London Her Majesty Stationary Office.

Help the Aged (2002) Age Discrimination in Public Policy: A Review of Evidence: London: Help the Aged.

(http://www.tunstall.co.uk/Our-products/Telecare-solutions/ Individual-homes)..

Hood, C (1991), A Public Management for all seasons? Public Administration, 69 (1) pp 3-19.

Hudson, B (2002) Interprofessionlityin Health and Social Care: the Achilles' heel of partnership, Journal of Interprofessional Care, 16, 6, pp.15-34

Hughes, B (1995). Older People and Community Care, Buckingham Press. Open University.

Human Rights Act (1998): European Convention of Human Rights. London. Her Majesty Stationary Office.

Hunter, S and Ritchie, P (2007) Co-production and Personalisation in Social Care: Changing Relationships in the Provision of Social Care, London: Jessica Kinsley Publishers.

Joseph Rowntree Foundation (2009) Finding out What Determines " a Good Life" for Older People in Care Homes. Joseph Rownetree Foundation. York.

Joseph Rowntree Foundation (2007) Elderly Abuse: Joseph Rowntree Foundation. York

Joseph Rowntree Foundation (1994) Improving Older people in Community Care Planning. Research findings: 55 York: Joseph Rowentree Foundation.Jutras, S & Veilleux, F (1991): Informal Care giving: Correlates of Perceived Burden. Canadian Journal of Ageing 10, 40-55.

Kavanagh, D and Sildon, A (1999) The Power Behind the prime Minister, London: Harper Collins.

Kendall J, Matosevic T, Forder J, Knapp, Hardy B, Ware P. (2003): The Motivations of Domiciliary Care Providers in England: Building a Typology. London: London School of Economics.

Kiernan, K and Wicks, M (1990): Family Change and Future Policy, York Joseph Rowntree Memorial Trust.

King's Fund (2005a): Understanding Public Services and Care Markets. London: King's Fund.

King's Fund (2006): Securing Good Care for Older People: Taking a Long-Term View. Wanless Social Care Review London: King's Fund.

Kreimer, M (2006) "Developments in Austrian Care Arrangements", in C Glendinning and P. A. Kemp (eds), Cash and Care: Policy challenges in the welfare state. Policy Press, Bristol.

Leadbeater, C (2004). Personalisation through Participation: A New Script for Public Services, London Demos.

Lee, G (1985): Kinship and Social Support: The Care of the United States, Ageing and Society 5 (4): 19-38.

Leece, J (2000): It's a Matter of Choice: Making Direct Payments Work in Staffordshire: Practice, Volume 12 no 4 pp 37-48.

Lefley, H. (2001). "Mental Health Treatment and Service Delivery in Cross-Cultural Perspective." In Cross-Cultural Topics in Psychology, ed. L. L. Adler and U. P. Gielen. Westport, CT: Praeger.

Lewis, J (2006a): Care and Gender; have the arguments for recognising care work now been won? In cash and care. Edited by Glendinning, C, Kemp, P. Polity Press.

Lewis, J (2006b): Gender and welfare in modern Europe: In the art of survival, gender and history in Europe, 1450-2000. Past and present supplement. Edited by Harris, R; Roper, L Oxford University Press.

Lewis, J (2006): Perceptions of risk in intimate relationships: the implications for social provision. Journal of Social Policy 35, no 1, pp39-57.

Lewis, J and Glennerster, H (1996): Implementing the New Community Care, Buckingham: Open University Press.

Lewis, J (2005) 'The Changing Context for the Obligation for care and to earn', in M. Maclean (ed) Family Law and Family Values, Oxford: Hart Publishing.

Lewis, J (2004): Gender, Work, Family and Welfare State: The Nordic Countries in Comparative perspective; in Research on the Study of the Nordic Welfare State: Papers from the August 2003 Conference Helsinki. 16. Edited by Marjanen, J; Stenius, H; Vauhkonen, J. Renvall Institute Publications, 2004.

Lewis, J (2003): Responsibilities and Rights: Changing the Balance. In Developments in British Social Policy 2 Edited by Ellison, N: Pierson, C; Palgrave.

Lewis, J (2002): Individualisation, Assumptions about the Existence of an Adult worker Model and the Shift towards Contractualism; in Analysing Families: Mortality and rationality in Policy and practice. Edited by Carling, A; Duncan, S; Edwards, R. Routledge .

Lister, R (2001). New Labour: a study in ambiguity from a position of ambivalence, Critical Social Policy, 21, 4 pp 425-47.

Lloyds, M (2002). Care Management in R. Adams, L Dominelli and M Payne eds, Critical Practice in Social work, Basingstoke Palgrave.

Lowe, R (2003): Welfare State in Britain since 1945, 3rd edn, London Palgrve

Lundh, U. (1999). "Family Carers: Sources of Satisfaction among Swedish Carers." British Journal of Nursing 8(10):647–652.

Lymbery, M (1998a). Care Management and Professional Autonomy: The Impact of Community Care Legislation on Social Work with Older people, British Journal of Social work, 28, 6 pp 863-78

Lymbery, M (1998b). Social Work in General Practice: Dilemmas and Solutions, Journal of Inter-professional Care 12, 2 pp 199-209.

Lymbery, M (2001). Social work in Crossroads, British Journal of Social Work 31, 3 pp 369-84.

Lymbery, M (2003). Collaborating for the Social and Health Care of Older People in L, Whittington, J, Weinstein and T, Leiba eds Collaboration in Social Work practice. London, Jessica Kingsley.

Lymbery, M (2004a). Managerialism and Care Management Practice, in M Lymbery and S, Butler eds, Social Work Ideals and Practice Realities, Basingstoke, Palgrave.

Lymbery, M (2004b). The Changing Nature of Welfare Organisation, in M Lymbery and, S Butler ed. Social Work Ideals and Practice Realities, Basingstoke, Palgrave.

Lymbery, M and Butler, S (2004). Social work Ideals and practice realities, Basingstoke, Palgrave.

Lymbery, M and Millward, A (2001). Community Care in Practice: Social Work in Primary Healthcare, Social Work in Healthcare, 34, 3 / 4 pp 241-59.

Lymbery, M (2004). Delayed Discharge: Preparing for Reimbursement, Journal of Integrated Care, 12, 4 pp 28-34.

Maglajcic, R, Brandon, D and Given, D (2000): Making the Direct Payments a Choice, a Report on the Research Findings. Disability and Society Volume 15 no 1 pp 99-13.

Machin, S and Waldfogel, J (1994): The decline of male breadwinner, STICERD, Welfare State Programme Discussion Paper WSP/103, London: London School of Economics.

McRae, S (1999) (eds) Changing Britain: Families and Households in the 1990s. Oxford: Oxford University Press.

Means, R, Smith, R (1998a): Community Care: Policy and Practice (2nd. Ed) Basingstoke: Macmillan.

Means, R and Smith, R (1995): The Development of Welfare Service for Elderly People, London: Groom Helm.

Mellor, D (2004): Employers Report Higher pay and better news on Retention, Community Care 29 (7)–4(8) 2004.

Milner, J and O'Byrne, P (2002) Assessment in Social Work (2nd ed) Basingstoke, Palgrave.

Moroney, R (1976): The Family and State. London. Longman.

Morris, J (1993a): Independent Lives: Community Care and Disabled People: Basingstoke: Macmillan.

Murray, J.; Scheider, J.; Banerjee, S.; and Mann, A. (1999). "Eurocare: A Cross-National Study of Co-Resident Spouse Carers for People with Alzheimer's Disease." International Journal of Geriatric Psychiatry 14(8):662–667.

Noelker, L. S., and Bass, D. M. (1994). "Relationships between the Frail Elderly's Informal and Formal Helpers." In Family Care giving across the Lifespan, ed. E.

Organisation for Economic Co-operations and Developments (2005) Long-Term Care for Older People, OECD, Paris.

Organisation for Economic Co-operations and Developments (1988): Ageing Populations: The Social Policy Implications, Paris, OECD.

Organisation for Economic Co-operations and Developments (1998): The Employment Outlook, Paris. OECD.

O'Hara, G (2004): "We Are Faced Everywhere With a Growing Population". Demographic Change and the British State, 1945-64, Twentieth Century British History Vol, 15, no 3, pp 243-66.

Office of Population Census and Survey (1995/1996): General Household Surveys. London: Stationary Office

Office for National Statistics (2001) Living in Britain, WWW.Statistics. gov.uk, accessed 28 June 2004.

Oliver, M (1990) The politic of Disability, London: Mcmillian.

Olson, L. K., ed. (1994). The Graying of the World: Who Will Care for the Frail Elderly. New York: Haworth Press.

Osborne, D and Gaebler, T (1992) Reinventing Government: How the Entrepreneurial spirit is transforming the public sector (Reading MA: Addison-Wesley).

Payne, M (2000). The Politics of Case Management and Social Work, International Journal of Social Welfare, 9, 2 pp 82-91.

Pearson, C (2004a). Keeping the cash under control: What are the problems with Direct Payments in Scotland? Disability and Society, Vol 19, No 1 pp3-14.

Pearson, C (2004b). The Implementation of Direct Payments: Issues for user-led organizations in Scotland, in Barnes, C and Mercer, G (eds) (2004) Implementing the Social Models of Disability: Theory and Research, Leeds: Disability Press.

Pearson, C (2006). Developments in Direct Payments, Bristol: Policy Press.

Phillips J. Ray M. Ogg J. (2003) 'Exploring Conflict and Ambivalence' in Lowenstein A et al 'Old Age and Autonomy: The role of Service Systems and Intergenerational Family Solidarity' Final Report.

Phillips J. Ray M. Ogg J. (2003) 'Ambivalence et conflict dans les families vieillissantes: perspectives europeenes' Retraite en Societe

Phillips J Ray M and Marshall M (2006) 'Social Work with Older People' Hampshire, Palgrave.

Phillipson.C, Barnard. M and Strang. P, (1986): Dependency and Politics 19 (1): 27 – 36.

Phillipson, C (1990): Intergenerational relations: Conflict or Consensus in the Twenty First Century, Policy and Interdependency in old age. London: Croom Helm.

Phillipson, C, Burrand, M, Phillips, J, and Ogg (2001); The Family and Community Life of Older People: Household Composition and Social Networks in three Urban Areas: Ageing and Society 18 pp 259 –90.

Pickard L, Wittenberg R. Comas-Herrera A, Davis B. and Darton B. (2000): Relying on Informal care in the new century. Informal care for elderly people in England to 2031, Ageing and Society 20(6): 745-772.

Postle, K (2002) "Working Between the Idea and the Reality", Ambiguities and Tensions in Care managers Work, British Journal of Social Work.

Powell, M (2002). New Labour and the Third Way in the British Welfare State: a new and distinctive approach, Critical Social Policy, 20, 1 pp 30-60.

Powell, M A and Hewitt, M (1998): The end of the Welfare State, Social Policy and Administration, Vol 32 pp 1-13.

Quereshi, H and Walker, A (1998): The Caring Relationship: Elderly People and their Families, London. Macmillan.

Qureshi, H Patmore, C, Nicholas, E and Bumford (2002): Outcome of social care for older people and carers: social policy research unit. University of York England.

Qureshi, H and walker, A (1989) The Caring Relationships. London: Macmillan.

Ray M (2000) 'Older Women, Long Term Marriage and Care' in Bernard M. Phillips J. Machin L. Harding Davies V. (eds) Women Ageing: Changing Identities, Challenging Myths'.

Ray M and Phillips J (2002) 'Older People' in Adams R. Dominelli L. Payne M. (eds) Critical Practice in Social Work' Palgrave.

Ray M (2006) 'Informal Care in the context of long term marriage: The challenge to practice' in Practice 18(2) pp 129-142 .

Ray M (2007) 'Redressing the Balance; the participation of older people in research' in Bernard, M and Scharf T (in press) 'Critical perspectives on ageing societies ' Policy Press .

Raynes N., Clark H., Beecham J. (eds) (2006): Evidence submitted to the Older People's Inquiry into 'That Little Bit of Help". York: Joseph Rowntree Foundation.

Raynes, N, Temple, B, Glenister, C, Coultherd, L (2001) Getting Older People's Views on Quality Home Care Services. Joseph Rownetree Foundation. York.

Riddell, S, Pearson, C, Barnes, C, Jolly, D, Mercer, G and Priestley, M (2005). The Developments of Direct Payments in the UK: Implications for Social Justice, Social Policy and society, Vol 4, No1 PP 75-85.

Roberts, E (1995) Women and Family: An Oral History 1940-1970. Oxford: Blackwell.

Rosser, C and Harris, C, C (1965) The family and social Change. London: Routledge.

Royal Commission on Long Term Care (1999): With Respect to Old Age. Report of the Royal Commission on the Funding of Long Term Care for the Elderly, London HMSO.

Sale, A and Leason, K (2004): Is help easily at hand? Direct Payment: Community Care Journal 6-12 pp 28-31 May 2004.

Scruton, R (1980): The Meaning of Conservatism. Harmondsworthy. Penguin.

Tessler, R., and Gamache, G. (2000). Family Experiences with Mental Illness. Westport, CT: Auburn House.

Thane, P (2000): Old Age in English History: Past Experiences, Present Issues, Oxford: Oxford University Press.

Townsend, P (1983): A Theory of Parents and the Role of Social Policy in Joney et al (1983).

Twigg, J (2006) The Body in Health and Social Care, London: Palgrave.

Twigg, J and Atkin, K (1994) Carers' Perceived Policy and Practice in Informal Care, Buckingham: Open University Press.

Ugwumadu. A U. (2010) Unpublished Doctoral thesis. Family Directed Support Care Systems: Anglia Ruskin University, UK

United Nations Organisation (1999): World Population Prospects: The 1998 Review, Vol 1: Comprehensive Tables, New York: UN.

United Nations Organisation (1982): Report of the World Assembly on ageing. Vienna, 26 July to 6 August. UNO, New York.

United Nations Organisation (2002): Report of the second World Assembly on Ageing. UNO, New York.

Walker, A (1995): The Family and the Mixed Economy of Care. Can they be integrated? In I Allen and E Perkins (Eds) The Future of Family Care for Older People, London: HMSO.

Walker, M (1998): The Third Way International, New Statesmen 27 March pp 30-2.

Wanless Report (2006): The future of social care funding. HMSO: Reference number 2006/0121.

Webb, A and Weston, G (1982): The Personal Social Services: Expediency, Instrumentalism or Systematic Social Planning, London: Heinemann.

Wellman, B and Wortley, S (1989): Brothers Keepers: Situational Kinship Relations in Broader Networks of Social Support: Sociological Perspectives 32- pp 273 – 306.

Wiener, J , Tilly, J and Cuellar, A. E (2003) Consumer-directed Home Care in the Netherlands, England and Germany, AARP Public Policy Institute, Washington DC.

Wilkinson, H (2000) The Family Business. London: Demos.

Wilkinson, H (1999) Celebrate the New Family. New Statesman, 9th August.

Wilkinson, H (1998) The Family Way: Navigating a third way in family policy, in Tomorrow's Politics: The Third Way and beyond, ed. Ian Hargreaves and Ian Christie, 112-25, London Demos.

Wistow G. (2005): Developing Social Care: the past, the present, the future, London: SCIE.

Wistow, G, and Hardy, B (1998): Domiciliary Care: Mission Accomplished? Policy and Politics 24.2.

Wistow, G, Herbert, G, Townsend, J, Ryan, J, Wright, D, Ferguson, B (2002b): Rehabilitation Pathway for Older People after Fractured Neck of Femur: Executive Survey, Leeds: Nuffield Institute for Health.

Wistow, G, Waddingham, E, Fong Cheu, L (2002a): Intermediate Care: Burdening the System, Leeds: Nuffield Institute for Health.

World Bank (1994): Averting the old age crisis. Oxford University Press, Oxford.

World Health Organisation (1989): Health of the elderly Report,

Young, R, Hardy, B, and Wistow, G (1999): Who's choice? How Users, Carer and Care Managers see the Assessment and Care Management System, Evidence. Briefing Paper 4, Personal Social Service Unit, London School of Economics and Nuffield Institute for Health, University of Leeds.

Young, M and Willmott, P (1957) Family and kinship in East London: London: Routledge and Kegan Paul.

Zarb, G and Nadash, P (1994). Cashing in on Independence: Comparing the costs and Benefits of Cash and Services, London: BCODP.

Policy framework for end of life care for older people

This book is intended to have a wide UK and international audience. The book is aimed at policy makers, social work practitioners, researchers, service users and family caregivers in the UK and the English speaking countries outside the United Kingdom. It is intended also for use on professional training courses for Nursing, Occupational Therapy, Social Work, and Health Visitors for Adult and Older People service users. Given the large number of practitioners across a range of disciplines, the author is confident that there will be a considerable demand for the book with regard to the Modernisation of Services, the changing Demography and the Big Society agenda.

About the author and Qualifications

The author is a Gerontologist currently employed by Essex County Council as an operational manager within the Adult Social Care and Community Well-being Department. Prior to this employment, his experience stretched over twenty five years working at various levels in five different Social Services Departments in the UK. He is also a qualified Health and Social Care professional with many years experience in National Health Services. In both Health and Social Care, his professional practices centred on older people services for which he desired to make contributions to knowledge as a specialist in the sector. During this period, his knowledge has been developed with his continuous professional and academic studies at various universities in the UK and he gained his Doctorate Degree in Health and Social Care Policy.

FELIX. U. A. UGWUMADU